Nursing Care in a Violent Society

Harriet R. Feldman, PhD, RN, is Dean and Professor of Nursing at Pace University's Lienhard School of Nursing. She is one of the Founding Editors of *Scholarly Inquiry for Nursing Practice*, Assistant Editor for Research of the *Journal of Professional Nursing,* and a member of the Editorial Advisory Board of the *Journal of the New York State Nurses Association.* She has been recognized for her contributions by her recent selection for fellowship in the American Academy of Nursing. Dr. Feldman's strong commitment to nursing science is reflected in her research, writings, and presentations, and her active involvement in professional organizations. As Editor of *Nursing's Response to Our Culture of Violence,* she further supports this commitment.

NURSING CARE *IN A* VIOLENT SOCIETY

Issues and Research

Harriet R. Feldman, PhD, RN
Editor

Springer Publishing Company

Copyright © 1995 by Springer Publishing Company, Inc.

All rights reserved

No part of this publication may be reproduced, stored in a retrieval system, or transmitted, in any form or by any means, electronic, mechanical, photocopying, recording, or otherwise, without the prior permission of Springer Publishing Company, Inc.

Springer Publishing Company, Inc.
536 Broadway
New York, NY 10012

Cover design by Tom Yabut
Production Editor: Pam Ritzer

95 96 97 98 99 / 5 4 3 2 1

Library of Congress Cataloging in Publication Data

Nursing care in a violent society: issues and research / Harriet R. Feldman, editor.
    p. cm.
    "Derived from a special issue of *Scholarly Inquiry for Nursing Practice: An International Journal"* —Intro.
    Includes bibliographical references and index.
    ISBN 0-8261-9080-4
    1. Nursing—Social aspects—United States. 2. Violence—United States. 3. Violence—United States—Prevention. 4. Violence—United States—Health aspects. 5. Victims of family violence—United States. I. Feldman, Harriet R. II. Scholarly inquiry for nursing practice.
    [DNLM: 1. Nursing—United States. 2. Violence—United States. 3. Social Conditions—United States. WY 300 AA1 N93 1995]
    RT86.5.N87 1995
    610.73—dc20
    DNLM/DLC   95-31624
    for Library of Congress   CIP

Printed in the United States of America

Contents

Contributors	*vii*
Introduction: Nursing's Response to our Culture of Violence Harriet R. Feldman	*ix*

1 An Overview of Violence in America and Nursing's
   Response: Demographics, Research, and Public Policy   1
   Jacquelyn C. Campbell, Mary J. Harris,
   and Roberta K. Lee

2 Battered Women's Anxiety for Their Children:
   A Study   23
   Janice Humphreys

3 Toward Effective Treatment of Abused Women:
   What Nurses Can Do   43
   Marylou Yam

4 Preventing Child Abuse and Neglect Through Home
   Visitation: Hawaii's Healthy Start Program   55
   Vicki A. Wallach and Larry Lister

5 The Psychological Impact of Caring for Victims
   of Violence: Vicarious Traumatization   71
   Carol Hartman

6 Ethical Problems in Caring for Violent
   Psychiatric Patients   89
   Anastasia Fisher

Index   *105*

Contributors

Jacquelyn C. Campbell, RN, PhD
Professor
College of Nursing
Johns Hopkins University
Baltimore, MD 21218

Anastasia Fisher, RN, DNSc
University of San Francisco
San Francisco, CA 94117

Mary J. Harris, RN, DrPH
Assistant Professor
School of Nursing
University of Texas Medical
Branch at Galveston
Galveston, TX 77555

Carol R. Hartman, RN, CS, DNSc
Boston College
School of Nursing
Chestnut Hill, MA 02167

Janice Humphreys, PhD, RN, CS
Department of Family Health Care
Nursing
University of California,
San Francisco
San Francisco, CA 94143

Roberta K. Lee, RN, DrPH
Professor
School of Nursing
University of Texas Medical
Branch at Galveston
Galveston, TX 77555

Larry Lister, DSW
University of Hawaii – Manoa
Honolulu, HI 96822

Vicki A. Wallach
Child and Family Service
200 N. Vineyard Boulevard
Honolulu, HI 96817

Marylou Yam, PhD, RN
Assistant Professor
St. Peter's College
Jersey City, NJ 07306

vii

Introduction:
Nursing's Response to our
Culture of Violence

I am neither victim nor perpetrator. I live in a predominantly white, middle-class, suburban neighborhood with my husband and two college-age children. While encounters with face to face violence during my life have been rare, I am confronted daily by a stream of violence reported in print, sight, and sound. I cannot help but be affected by these reports of individual, family, and societal violence. As someone who interacts with the health care system, both as a consumer and health professional, I am acutely aware of the overwhelming need to reframe the thinking and actions of all health professionals to address what has become a problem of epidemic proportions — a culture of violence.

This culture affects women, children, elders, and families, but it also invades the once trusted systems of everyday life, for example, our schools and hospitals. It is a social "disease" of epidemic proportions (Deborah Prothrow-Stith, 1994). The statistics are startling: "every six minutes, somewhere in this country, a woman is raped and every 15 seconds a woman will be beaten" ("Violence against Women," 1991, p. 6); in 1993, 1300 abused children died (Ingrassia & McCormick, 1994). A University of Michigan study estimated that about 270,000 guns are present in school every day (Cassetta, 1994); homicide is the leading cause of death for young black men and for infants between 6 weeks and 2 years of age (AAN Working Paper, 1993); elder abuse affects between 700,000 and 1,000,000 men and women annually (AAN Working Paper, 1993); and reports of assault by patients in psychiatric units and emergency rooms are escalating (Morton, 1987; "Nurses under the Gun," 1994). The streets of our cities are a backdrop for crime. A special report in *Newsweek* ("A Week in the Death of America," 1993) described a week of death in America, reviewing a week of homicides in 10 cities. Also reported were the number of homicides by year in five-year intervals since 1970. With the exception of 1985 (18,980 homicides), the number of homicides has consistently risen from 16,000 in 1970 to an estimated 24,500 in 1993. The toll, however, reaches beyond the criminals and victims. It reaches "beyond the crime scenes and into the communities where the impact of murder reverberates daily" ("A Week in the Death of America," 1993, p. 24).

There are political and economic parameters that keep violence in the forefront. In a July 17, 1994, Op-Ed article in the *New York Times*, Herbert writes about a 9-year-old who was killed on the streets of New Orleans walking home from a picnic on Mother's Day. He tells how this boy had written to President Clinton asking that he "stop the killing in the city" (Herbert, 1994, p. E17), and how different his life was when he was 9 years-old. Herbert writes, "When I was nine the only thing I worried about was Willie Mays' batting average. It couldn't have occurred to me that I might die. On the street in the summer my friends and I listened for the tinkling of the ice cream truck, not an explosion of gunfire. The sound we dreaded most was of our parents calling us inside. Drastic changes in values have occurred since then. And some of those changes have enabled us to accept the wholesale destruction of American children as more or less routine" (p. E17). These values are reinforced because they perpetuate the separation of the unaffected "we" and the affected "them." The economic gains of violence are a force as well. The penal system is big business—a high-growth industry. For example, Cronin (1994) discusses the price of a death penalty sentence, citing that "the average cost to try a noncapital murder case and keep a criminal in prison for 20 years" (p.3) is $166,000 and "the average cost to try, convict, and execute a murderer" (p.3), including a lengthy appeals process, is $329,000. While we have reduced defense expenditures in this country and are experiencing decreasing funding for education, we have at the same time increased the dollars spent on the construction and operation of prisons.

Domestic violence is a widespread problem that crosses cultural, racial, socioeconomic, religious, gender, and age groups, and affects families, communities, and larger systems. Recognition of the problem beyond the home is relatively recent. The first shelter for battered women opened in 1974; just 20 years later, there were 20,000 programs in the United States for battered women (Diamond, 1994). Innovative programs give evidence of beginning recognition in the legal community. For example, the Battered Women's Justice Center at Pace University, the only such program in the United States, was formed by New York State and Pace University in 1991 to teach lawyers how to handle domestic violence cases.

Domestic violence impacts beyond the principals involved, as evidenced in one study where 70% of teenagers in jail for homicide witnessed their mothers being abused (Diamond, 1994). The legislative playing field is also changing. For example, the April 6, 1994, edition of *Newsday* (Katz, 1994) reported that a Massachusetts state court invoked civil rights laws in a domestic violence case, stating that the "man accused of battering women was probably motivated by hatred or bias against women as a class" (p.17). Both United States Senate and House of Representatives crime bills include the Violence Against Women Act "for programs to combat domestic violence. One proposal in the Senate bill would allow women to use civil-rights violations as a basis to seek

Introduction   xi

damages against their assailants" (Katz, 1994, p.17). In addition, the Family Protection and Domestic Violence Intervention Act of 1994 "requires mandatory arrest of batterers who violate orders of protection or commit a felony assault against the victim ("Domestic Violence," 1994, p.11).

This book, derived from a special issue of *Scholarly Inquiry for Nursing Practice: An International Journal* focuses on nursing's response to our "culture of violence." It begins with an overview of violence epidemiology and research, prevention approaches, and policy implications. In the lead chapter, Jacquelyn Campbell, Mary Harris, and Roberta Lee provide a context for us to consider the magnitude and dynamics of our culture of violence, including national data sources and outcomes of violence research conducted by nurses, and theories of family violence that form the basis for understanding child, spouse, and elder abuse. Equally important is the unique orientation of the discipline of nursing, characterized by the authors as avoiding "much of the victim blaming and emphasis on pathology characteristic of other disciplines, research which has viewed women victimized by violence as a deviant group" (p. 18). This perspective, in addition to guiding the actual research on violence conducted by nurses, directs the prevention approaches that nurses use, especially the creation and use of surveillance systems, conduct of research and program evaluation, implementation of injury prevention strategies, development of coalitions among organizations, and coordination of efforts to effect funding and legislation. The chapters that follow this overview concern themselves with the effects of violence on families (Humphreys), strategies for addressing wife (Yam) and child (Wallach & Lister) abuse, and the problems affecting nurses who care for (Hartman) or are themselves victims (Fisher) of violence.

Janice Humphreys conducted an ethnographic study concerning battered women's worries about their children. The 25 women interviewed had left abusive relationships and were living with their children in a shelter. Through interviews and participant observation, data were collected about these women's worries and their responses to the worries. While many of the worries described were typical of mothers in general, and some of the worries were more common to urban settings, others were unique, either in type or extent, to their specific circumstances. The major themes of "keeping your children safe" and "creating order out of disorder" arose out of past circumstances surrounding the abusive relationship, present circumstances in the shelter setting, and the anticipated future for their children. A cogent point made by Humphreys is that the violence these families experienced is reflective of the national violence that exists and is tolerated. She advocates for individuals and society to engage in interventions that prevent violence at every level and to all those at risk.

Marylou Yam's research on nurses who care for wife-abuse victims in the emergency room setting raises concerns about how the health care system responds to wife-abuse victims and what impedes a therapeutic response on the part of nurses. Her chapter on wife abuse focuses on these concerns as well as effective strategies for nursing intervention. Among the reasons for the type of response by health professionals are beliefs in stereotypes and cultural beliefs about women; the legitimacy of the problem; and the futility associated with attempts at change.

Particularly, Yam addresses the medical model as an interfering rather than facilitating force for change, viewing the medical model as one that promotes passivity of the victim and cure of the symptoms rather than their underlying cause. General use of this model by health professionals, she claims, has fostered continued dependence by victims on abusive relationships and the health delivery system instead of empowering abuse victims to break the cycle of violence. A great deal is still unknown about what constitutes an effective, helping nurse–patient relationship in situations where patients are victims of abuse; Yam argues for continued research to explicate this relationship.

Vicki Wallach and Larry Lister present a statewide model of child abuse prevention, Hawaii's Healthy Start program, that uses home visitation over an extended period of time to assist in the development of appropriate parenting behaviors, and to expand knowledge regarding ways to access health care. The home visitation program is based in a network of health care agencies, including hospitals and social service agencies within communities throughout the state. While basic services are alike, the culture of each agency can manifest its unique focus. Wallach and Lister report that the program is available to serve about half of Hawaii's families with newborns.

The success of the program is laudable. In a 1985 demonstration project involving 241 at-risk families, no cases of abuse and only four cases of neglect were found; data on 2254 families seen between July 1987 and July 1991 confirmed child abuse in only 16 families and neglect in about 30. Also impressive is that 90% of 2-year-olds were immunized, 85% of the children were developmentally age appropriate, and 95% of all children had an identified primary health care provider. These initial outcomes are most promising. I can't help but wonder about the long-range outcomes of Healthy Start, as these children reach adolescence and adulthood. For example, will there be a lower incidence of violence in the lives of these individuals as compared with the general population of Hawaii and the United States? The potential of this program to change our culture of violence seems great.

The remaining chapters address the experience of the provider as the victim of violence, including the emotional trauma and ethical problems encountered by nurses. Carol Hartman poses a concern not widely known, that of nurses' reactions to the trauma information shared by their patients in the context of the nurse–patient relationship. These reactions, expressed as symptoms of vicarious traumatization, both traumatize the nurse and negatively affect the therapeutic relationship. Nurses also experience feelings of guilt and inad-

Introduction   xiii

equacy because they cannot meet their role expectations while they are themselves traumatized. Through examples of nurse-patient encounters, Hartman develops the framework for understanding the nurse's countertransference reactions of avoidance or overidentification within the context of factors within the nurse, patient, and environment. As the nurse's capacity to be empathic is challenged, her/his reactions toward the patient become nontherapeutic. Institutional and professional support are critical if the nurse is to overcome the emotional response to working with victims of violence and resolve the role dilemmas that prevent successful patient encounters.

Anastasia Fisher addresses the difficulties of working with dangerous mentally ill patients. Psychiatric nurses experience a great deal of conflict in trying to be therapeutic and, at the same time, maintain control of violent behavior in the institutional setting. The balance is delicate and fraught with ethical dilemmas that need to be confronted and resolved. In her study of psychiatric nurses, Fisher identified three ethical problems: balancing support for patient autonomy with the need to maintain control (unit safety), balancing the need for distancing (personal safety) with the desire to establish therapeutic relationships, and balancing the desire to do the right thing with the need to get along with colleagues (image of self as nurse). These conditions make it extremely difficult to establish and nurture relationships in psychiatric nursing practice, whether they be with patients or colleagues. Furthermore, they serve to reinforce within the institution the culture of violence and make it impossible to maintain the values associated with caring. Finally, Fisher points out that we must consider these ethical problems if we are to create humane environments for patients and practitioners alike.

While this book gives us a sense of nurses' encounters with violence and identifies useful strategies for prevention, some important issues remain. Campbell, Harris, and Lee begin a discussion of policy implications for the discipline of nursing, focusing on the ability of nurses to influence policy development and the development of a research agenda that includes empowering the victims of violence. Yet there are broader, more far-reaching implications that affect us all. Nurses need to ask the "bigger" questions: Who benefits from violence? What are the political and economic payoffs? Why does violence continue? How can we change the values that have allowed us to tolerate or ignore the pain and move on? As nurses on the "front lines," we must take a leadership role in prevention, as prevention is our only hope for eliminating what Herbert (1994) refers to as "a moral abomination." We hope that this book, derived from a special issue of *Scholarly Inquiry,* stimulates you to confront these important questions and become active in changing the values and behaviors of our culture of violence, through research, teaching, clinical practice, and community service.

REFERENCES

AAN Working Paper–Violence as a nursing priority: Policy implications. (1993, March/April). *Nursing Outlook,* 41(2), 83-92.

A crime as American as a colt .45. (1994, August 15). *Newsweek,* 22-23.

A week in the death of America. (1994, August 15). *Newsweek,* 24-50.

Cassetta, R. A. (1994, April). Nurses work to prevent violence in schools. *The American Nurse,* 26(4), 7.

Cronin, A. (1994, December 4). Execution and murder: Looking hard at America's deadly numbers game. *The New York Times,* E1, 3.

Diamond, K. (1994, April 21). Society's role in stopping domestic violence. *Staten Island Advance,* Lifestyle Section, C2.

Domestic violence targeted. (1994, July 13). *Bellmore Life,* p. 11.

Herbert, B. (1994, July 17). Dear Mr. President. *The New York Times,* E17.

Ingrassia, M., & McCormick, J. (1994, April 24). Why leave children with bad parents? *Newsweek,* 52-58.

Katz, N. L. (1994, April 6). Domestic violence precedent. *Newsday,* A17.

Morton, P. G. (1987, August). Staff roles and responsibilities in incidents of patient violence. *Archives of Psychiatric Nursing,* 1(4), 280-284.

Nurses under the gun: Escalating violence prompts demand for new hospital safeguards. (1994, September). *Report,* 25(8), 1, 12.

Prothrow-Stith, Leader in Violence Prevention, to Speak on December 1. (1994, November 30). *The Delphian,* p. 3.

Violence against Women: Report of the June 21, 1991, Conference (1991, June 21). Conference Proceedings. *National Women's Health Resource Center,* Washington, DC, 80 pp.

1

An Overview of Violence in America and Nursing's Response: Demographics, Research, and Public Policy

Jacquelyn C. Campbell, Mary J. Harris, and Roberta K. Lee

This chapter discusses the problem of violence in America and presents an overview of pertinent research studies. It considers data sources on violence and the categorization of injuries. It next focuses on the specific problems of family violence: child abuse, spouse abuse, and elder abuse. The second part of the chapter considers the nursing discipline's specific contribution to violence research by reviewing nursing studies on abuse during pregnancy, female partner abuse, elder abuse, and child abuse. Nursing research, which is grounded in the clinical concerns of the discipline, is presented as having an advocacy orientation that avoids the victim blaming and emphasis on pathology often characteristic of other disciplines' research. The chapter discusses how nurses can participate in prevention approaches to reduce violence-related injuries, and it concludes by offering policy recommendations for nursing organizations.

During the past 10 years, violence has been identified as a public health problem as well as a criminal justice problem (Moore, 1993). Although the definition of violence in public health includes attempted suicide and suicide, the National Research Council's definition of violence only includes behaviors by individuals that intentionally threaten, attempt, or inflict physical harm on others (National Research Council, 1993b). Using this definition, in 1992, there were more than 22,000 homicides in the United States (U.S. Department of Justice, 1993), and more than 33,000,000 people reported other criminal victimizations, including nearly 2,000,000 physical injuries (U.S. Department of Justice, 1994). Injuries due to violence exact a tremendous toll on our country's health care, law enforcement, and criminal justice systems. The attention to violence by public health professionals brings a different perspective to the study of violence. Using the methods of epidemiology, public health professionals are studying how primary prevention strategies can reduce violence, whereas the criminal justice system has largely focused on secondary and tertiary preventions.

1

2   Nursing Care in a Violent Society: Issues and Research

DATA SOURCES

At a national level, the public health and criminal justice systems each collect information about violence. In public health, the national death registration system has included external cause codes (E-codes) on death certificates for many years. There is no parallel system, however, to identify nonfatally injured people. For some years, the national Centers for Disease Control and Prevention (CDC) have recommended adding E codes to the national hospital discharge data (Sniezek, Finklia, & Graitcek, 1989), but these data exclude people whose injuries are not serious enough to require hospitalization and people whose injuries are psychological. Developing surveillance systems for nonfatal injuries remains a challenge in public health.

There are two sources for violence data in the criminal justice system. The first is the Uniform Crime Reporting (UCR) system which is compiled from a uniform set of data collected by local police departments, representing 97% of the country. The uniform crime report for homicides is augmented by a standardized supplemental homicide report. Unfortunately, the data from the supplemental investigations are often not appended to the UCR system.

A second reporting system is the National Crime Victimization Survey (NCVS). The NCVS is a large, continuous random sample of households that are interviewed every six months. The survey, which uses a rolling-panel-survey design, includes only people over 12 years of age, and it excludes "victimless" crimes, such as drug abuse or prostitution. It is of interest that respondents to the NCS state that they have reported less than 40% of criminal victimizations to police.

It is clear that we do not yet have a single national source of data to measure the true magnitude of violence in our country. The available data systems yield different numbers, particularly for homicides and other serious crimes. For example, the national death registration system consistently reports 10% more homicides than the uniform crime reports, and the percentage has been increasing (CDC, 1992).

CATEGORIZATIONS OF INJURIES

One approach to injury classification is to classify all injuries according to the injury agent. Agents of injury are forms of energy—chemical, thermal, or mechanical—(Haddon, 1980). In this classification, it is possible to measure the impact of one type of injury—for example, a mechanical injury such as a firearm injury—by aggregating these injuries across all injury circumstances.

Firearm injuries provide a useful example of the impact of one type of injury. In the United States, more than 38,000 people died in 1991 due to the discharge of firearms (National Center for Health Statistics, 1993). A number

An Overview of Violence   3

of recent studies have evaluated the role of firearms in the home and the risks and benefits associated with their possession. Kellermann and Reay (1986) noted that for every case of firearm homicide attributed to self-protection, there were 1.3 unintentional homicides, 4.6 other homicides, and 33 firearm suicides. Lee and others (Lee, Waxweiller, Dobbins, & Paschetag, 1991) found that for each case of self-protection firearm injury, there were 108 other firearm injuries to people, usually family members and people known to the gun owner. Kellermann et al. (1993) found that the independent risk associated with keeping firearms in the home was 2.7-fold.

More commonly, injuries are subcategorized according to the intent of the injury, that is, homicide, suicide, or unintentional injury—or by the relationship between the "victim" and "offender," for example, spouse abuse—or by the age of the victim—child abuse, elder abuse. Interpretation of the findings of these often descriptive analyses can only be done by carefully considering who is eligible to be included in the case definition. For example, when prevalence studies of violence against pregnant women are conducted in prenatal clinics, the findings usually do not tell us whether the risk of domestic violence increases during pregnancy. In the next sections we present the findings of studies using the categorizations of homicide and family violence.

HOMICIDE

Homicide is the leading cause of death among black males and females ages 15–34; in this age group, it is the fourth leading cause of death among white females and third among white males (CDC, 1992). Homicides claim more lives than any other cause of death in the first year of life (Waller, Baker, & Szocka, 1989). More than half of homicide victims are killed by family members and most assailants are males. In most homicides, the victim and assailant are of the same race. Homicide is a particularly American problem, as our rates exceed those reported by every developed nation (Fingerhut & Kleinman, 1989). More than 60% of homicides are committed with firearms, followed by sharp instruments or knives (20%) and strangulation (5%) (Baker, O'Neill, Ginsburg, & Guohua, 1992). The majority of homicides occur in the home, though at least 600 homicides occur annually at work (Klaus, 1987). The rate of homicides for people living in central cities is about three times as high as the rate for people living elsewhere.

FAMILY VIOLENCE

We like to think of the American home as a place of safety and support, but for all too many people, it is no longer a "safe haven" against a violent society.

4   *Nursing Care in a Violent Society: Issues and Research*

Family violence has increased dramatically over the last 20 years, even though it is believed that intrafamily violence is substantially underreported because of the privacy surrounding family life. In 1990, intrafamily violence accounted for 18% of all homicides in the United States (FBI, 1991). While the overall risk of homicide for women is substantially lower than for men, the risk for women to be murdered by a family member is more than four times that of men (Kellermann & Mercy, 1992). The 1990 NCVS found that 6% of victims of violence were attacked by members of their own family, with two thirds of the attacks being assaults (Bureau of Justice Statistics, 1992). The type and severity of the assault differed by sex, age, and the victim-perpetrator relationship. Women suffered the most assaults; divorced, separated, and cohabiting women are at the greatest risk for assault. Younger children were more likely to be assaulted than older children, with females most often the perpetrators. Violence was also common between male members of the family.

There are three main theories or models that try to explain family violence. One theory emphasizes the psychopathology of the abuser (Gelles, 1974). The abuser is usually characterized as being mentally ill, developmentally disabled, or a substance abuser. This model assumes that violence has underlying behavioral or psychological causes.

In the family violence model, the root cause of family violence is thought to be violence learned in childhood, which is transmitted across generations (Straus, Gelles, & Steinmetz, 1980; Utech & Garrett, 1992). Victims of violence become perpetrators of violence. Kalmuss (1984) reports that a disproportionate number of wife abusers come from abusive families. Straus et al. (1980) found that women who were victims of severe violence at the hands of their spouses were 150% more likely to use severe violence to resolve conflicts with their children. In this "cycle of violence," the individual knows only one way to handle conflict—by force.

The third theory of family violence postulates that when stressful situations arise in the family (i.e., unemployment or the birth of a new baby), the perpetrator responds to the stress by directing violence at a family member (Pillemer & Finklehor, 1988). This theory assumes that violence arises among adults because they lack the skills to cope appropriately with stressful situations.

Child Abuse

Kempe, Silverman, Steele, Droegemuller, and Silver (1962) drew attention to the problem of child abuse and neglect with their article on the "battered child syndrome." The Child Abuse Prevention and Treatment Act, which was signed into law in 1974, established the National Center on Child Abuse and Neglect (NCCAN). The NCCAN has defined an abused or neglected child as "a child whose physical or mental health or welfare is harmed or threatened

An Overview of Violence   5

with harm by the acts or omissions of the child's parent or other person responsible for the child's welfare." While NCCAN's broad definition serves as the basis for current state laws on child maltreatment, it is not precise enough to use in research on the specific causes, nature, and extent of different types of child maltreatment (i.e., neglect, sexual abuse, physical abuse, emotional abuse).

There have been two national studies to determine the incidence of child abuse and neglect. The first, the National Incidence Study (NIS-1), was initiated in 1979, and a second study, the NIS-2, was conducted in 1986. Based on these studies, the NIS-1 (U.S. Department of Health & Human Services [USDHHS], 1981) estimated an overall incidence of child maltreatment of 9.8 cases per 1,000 children in 1980, which increased to 25.2 cases per 1,000 children in NIS-2 (USDHHS, 1988). Physical abuse was the most frequent type of abuse identified in the study (5.7 cases per 1000 children), followed by emotional abuse (3.4 cases per 1000 children), and sexual abuse (2.5 cases per 1000 children).

In 1988, NCCAN redesigned the child maltreatment data collection and analysis system. The 1990 information was collected from 49 states, one territory, Washington, DC, and the United States armed forces. There were 1.7 million reports of maltreatment, affecting 2.7 million children (National Research Council, 1993a).

Researchers generally agree that child maltreatment results from a complex interaction of individual, family, and environmental factors (Burgess & Draper, 1989). One consistent finding is that black children are more likely to be reported for child maltreatment than white children. NIS-2 reported that black children were one and one half times more likely to be physically abused than white children and five times more likely to die of physical abuse or neglect (USDHHS, 1988). NIS-2 also found that young children were at greater risk for both more serious and fatal injuries than older children. Several studies have found that children living in poverty are more likely to be reported for child abuse than higher income children (Gil, 1970; Hampton & Newberger, 1985).

It is also believed that the severity of the abuse increases with subsequent episodes. Sorenson and Peterson (1994) found child homicide victims were three times more likely than unintentional injury victims to have a documented history of child maltreatment before their deaths.

Interventions on behalf of victims of child maltreatment not only must help protect the child, but also include help for the family. The National Clinical Evaluation Study reported that the most cost-effective treatment plan for child sexual abuse is a combination of individual, group, and family counseling for the victim and the entire family (Daro, 1988). For child neglect, the study recommended family counseling, parent education, and the provision of basic services, such as babysitting, medical care, clothing, and housing. These treatment services can be costly, and the prevailing evidence suggests that treatment efforts are successful only in about one-half of families (Daro, 1988).

6   *Nursing Care in a Violent Society: Issues and Research*

Many child abuse researchers believe that primary prevention programs are the best way to reduce the incidence and impact of child maltreatment (Daro, 1988; National Research Council, 1993a). Programs that use nurses for prenatal and/or infancy home visits have shown promise in reducing the incidence of verified child abuse and neglect cases (Olds & Kitzman, 1990).

Spouse Abuse

Spouse abuse is usually defined as the use of physical force in intimate relationships among adults. In addition to physical battery, however, spouse abuse often encompasses a variety of behaviors, such as verbal threats, intimidating gestures, forced sexual activity, isolation, and economic deprivation (Okun, 1986). Spouse abuse usually applies to a wife who has been abused by her husband, but some studies have also reported husband abuse (Steinmetz, 1978). Abusive situations can also exist in homosexual relationships. Most states also have legal definitions for "domestic violence," which may not include all of the above behaviors.

The prevalence of spouse abuse is difficult to measure because of a woman's reluctance to identify her intimate partner as her abuser. Most authorities have estimated that from 20% to 40% of women have suffered abuse by their partners (Gin, Rucker, Frayne, Cygan, & Hubbell, 1991; "Shalala: Domestic abuse," 1994). According to a national representative study, 1.8 million wives are abused by their husbands each year (Straus & Gelles, 1986). In 1991, 5,745 women were victims of homicide, and about half of these women were killed by an intimate partner ("Shalala: Domestic abuse," 1994). Women are injured by abuse approximately 13 times as frequently as men (Stark & Flitcraft, 1991). Problems such as substance abuse, a history of violence, neglect, or sexual abuse in childhood or a personality profile that includes immaturity, hostility, an inability to communicate, lack of empathy, and low self-esteem are frequently found in perpetrators of spouse abuse (Gondolf & Foster, 1991; Stark & Flitcraft, 1991).

In addition to the three theories mentioned in our discussion of family violence, there is one additional theory that may apply to spouse abuse. The gender-politics model of spouse abuse suggests that violence in the family is part of a pattern of male control over females (Stark & Flitcraft, 1991). According to the gender-politics model, gender relations, rather than family dynamics, are responsible for spouse abuse. This model postulates that traditional male "machismo" attitudes evidence themselves through dating relationships, marriage, and parenting roles (Campbell & Fishwick, 1993). Men choose violence as a behavior when they feel that their control over their women is threatened.

While the physical injuries from assaults are a significant nursing issue, it is also important to treat the chronic health problems that are related to the

An Overview of Violence   7

experience of violence. For instance, the most common physical complaint of abused women is chronic pain (Goldberg & Tomlanovich, 1984). Irritable bowel syndrome, arthritis, and neurological damage, such as hearing loss, and other stress-related physical problems in women are also associated with years of physical assault from male partners (Campbell, 1989a; King & Ryan, 1989; Rodriguez, 1993). Chronic pelvic pain, sexually transmitted diseases, and pelvic inflammatory disease are common sequelae for women sexually abused in childhood and those raped in marriage (Campbell & Alford, 1989). Women with significant psychiatric illness, especially depression, posttraumatic stress disorder, and anxiety, are more likely to have a history of sexual and/or physical child or adult abuse than other women (Campbell, Smith-McKenna, Torres, Sheridan, & Landenburger, 1993).

Some 20% to 30% of emergency room visits by women are for injuries caused by domestic violence (Gin, Rucker, Frayne, Cygan, & Hubbell,1991; Goldberg & Tomlanovich, 1984). When women seek medical care for their injuries, health professionals have an opportunity to assess and diagnose abuse. Several studies done in health care settings, however, have found that women are infrequently asked about abuse. Hamberger, Saunders, and Hovey (1992) found that in a family practice clinic in the Midwest, 22.7% of the women attending the clinic had been physically assaulted by their partner within the last year, and 38.8% reported a lifetime pattern of physical abuse. Only six of these women, however, reported ever having a physician ask them about abuse.

Elder Abuse

One problem in studying elder abuse is that of definition. Researchers have identified a diverse range of problems as "elder abuse," including lack of proper housing, untreated medical conditions, and lack of social services. Phillips (1983) categorized 11 dimensions of elder abuse: physical abuse, physical neglect, emotional abuse, emotional neglect, emotional deprivation, sexual exploitation, verbal assault, medical neglect, material (financial) abuse, neglect of the environment, and violation of rights. Bristowe and Collins (1989) defined elder abuse as physical abuse, verbal abuse, passive neglect, and active neglect. In reality, many of the problems faced by the elderly are due more to neglect or the omission of an act, rather than the commission of an act of abuse. Furthermore, since elder abuse is of interest to a variety of health professionals, social workers, attorneys, and researchers, it is often defined differently to serve different purposes In 1992, the American Medical Association identified five classifications of elder abuse: physical or sexual abuse, psychological abuse, exploitation of assets, medical abuse (withholding necessary treatment), and neglect.

An additional problem in defining elder abuse lies in the lack of a uniform definition of who is "elderly." The U.S. Senate has created the following categories to classify older Americans: older population—age 55 to 64, elderly—age 65 to 74, aged—age 75-84, and the very old—85 years and over (U.S. Senate, 1983). As in the case of child abuse and neglect, the lack of specificity in the definition of elder abuse and neglect has made it difficult for researchers to generalize rates of maltreatment to the entire elder population, and to design effective intervention strategies.

Using age 65 or older as their definition of elderly, Pillemer and Finkelhor (1988) conducted a study of the scope and nature of maltreatment of the elderly occurring in the Boston metropolitan area. The study, a stratified random sample of 2,020 elderly persons, inquired about respondents' experiences with physical violence, chronic verbal aggression, and neglect by family members. The authors found that between 2.5% to 3.9% of the population had been maltreated in one or more of these areas. Applying that rate to the U.S. population would mean that between 701,000 and 1,093,560 elderly persons were abused. Since the definition of elder abuse in this study was not inclusive of all categories of abuse, this rate should be viewed as a minimum.

Studies have found that abused individuals tend to be female, disproportionately older (over age 75), show increased vulnerability due to an illness or impairment, and live with the perpetrator (Block & Sinnott, 1979; Shiferaw et al., 1994). The abuser is frequently one of the victim's own children, over the age of 40, female, and living in the same household (Pillemer & Frankel, 1991; Sengstock & Liang, 1983). The primary risk factor for elder abuse is that an adult child has been violent previously in another context (Pillemer & Finkelhor, 1988).

In addition to the aforementioned three theories of family violence, there are two theories based on dependency that apply to elder abuse. One theory emphasizes the caregiver stress as a risk factor for elder abuse (Cicirelli, 1983). Abuse results from the resentment generated by the increased dependency (financial, physical, and/or emotional) of an older, more impaired person on a caregiver. As the burdens increase for the caregiver, the caregiver may become abusive if he/she cannot cope with increased responsibilities. The second dependency theory pertains to abuser dependency on the abused. One study reported that abusers of the elderly were very dependent individuals who needed financial and other types of support from their victims (Pillemer & Finkelhor, 1988). For example, an adult child who is still dependent on an elderly parent for financial support may feel powerless and maltreat the parent.

Studies on the types of elder abuse have found different profiles for abuse, neglect, and financial exploitation (Wolf, 1994). Physical and psychological abuse were more related to problems of the perpetrator than the victim. Perpetrators were likely to have a history of psychopathology and to depend on the victim for financial assistance. Cases of neglect, on the other hand, seemed to be related to the dependency needs of the victims, who were often widowed, old, and impaired. Perpetrators in neglect cases found caring for the elderly a

An Overview of Violence   9

burden and a source of stress. In financial exploitation cases, greed was the apparent motivating factor. Victims were likely to be widows who were socially isolated. Perpetrators had financial problems and often had histories of substance abuse.

If elder abuse is thought to be primarily a result of caregiver stress, it is important to reduce that stress by providing respite care, meals-on-wheels, day care, and homemaker and aid services to the family. If the abuse is related to either the emotional or financial dependency of the perpetrator on the victim, treatment services for the perpetrator should include: vocational counseling, job placement, housing assistance, alcohol and drug treatment, mental health services, and financial support.

NURSING RESEARCH ON VIOLENCE

Nurses have always given excellent physical care to gunshot victims, battered women, sexual assault victims, and other victims of violence. Nurses have been part of the clinical team that has identified child abuse and cared for abused children. Nursing has contributed some of the earliest and most significant rape, wife, and elder abuse research of the health care disciplines (e.g., Burgess & Holstrom, 1974). This contribution has been both an important addition to the interdisciplinary knowledge base about violence and the basis for a distinct body of nursing knowledge about violence.

Abuse During Pregnancy

Perhaps the most significant contribution of accumulated nursing research on violence has been on the subject of abuse during pregnancy. The groundbreaking study by Helton, McFarlane, and Anderson (1987) of the prevalence of abuse during pregnancy was followed by the research of Judith McFarlane, Barbara Parker, Linda Bullock, and others, which significantly influenced nursing care in prenatal settings and related health care policy. Their research established a link between abuse during pregnancy and low birthweight and validated a four-question abuse screen, which is now widely recommended for use with *all* women entering the health care system (Bullock & McFarlane, 1989; Bullock, McFarlane, Bateman, & Miller, 1989). Although the screen can be used as a self-report series of questions on a nursing/health history form, significantly more women disclose abuse if asked questions by a nurse in an empathetic, private interview (Parker & McFarlane, 1991).

In a recent large prospective study of abuse during pregnancy, McFarlane and others (McFarlane, Parker, Soekin, & Bullock, 1992) found a 16% prevalence rate of abuse during the current pregnancy, the highest reported prevalence in all research on abuse during pregnancy. This high prevalence

10 *Nursing Care in a Violent Society: Issues and Research*

rate was thought to be related to the regular prenatal clinic nurse asking the questions during *each* regular prenatal visit. The researchers also discovered that abused women were significantly more likely to enter prenatal care in the third trimester, and they found that 24% of pregnant adolescents were physically and/or sexually abused during pregnancy (Parker, McFarlane, & Soeken, 1993). In another study of abuse during pregnancy, Campbell and associates (Campbell, Poland, Waller, & Ager, 1992) found that depression, anxiety, lack of social support, housing problems, and inadequate prenatal care were significant correlates with battering.

Female Partner Abuse

Other nursing research on wife abuse includes the finding that approximately 20% of women treated in emergency rooms have a history of abuse (Bullock, McFarlane, Bateman, & Miller, 1989; Goldberg & Tomlanovich, 1984; Helton, McFarlane, & Anderson, 1987). In spite of this high prevalence of abused women in prenatal and emergency settings, Brendtro and Bowker (1989) found that abused women rated health care professionals as the least helpful of all formal support system professionals. A more recent study of abused women who sought care in emergency departments (ED) found that problems in their care were related to race and poverty, as well as being abused (Campbell, Pliska, Taylor, & Sheridan, in press). The suggestions of these women have been incorporated into a model ED policy for domestic violence. Tilden and Shepherd (1987) have provided evidence of the effectiveness of an ED training program, but additional studies are needed.

Nursing research has consistently found low self-esteem in battered women, especially those that are also sexually abused (Campbell, 1989a; Campbell, 1989b; Trimpey, 1989; Ulrich, 1991; Weingourt, 1990). Both Weingourt (1990) and Campbell (1989b; Campbell & Alford, 1989) have contributed substantively to the knowledge that abused wives not only are frequently subjected to marital rape, but that rape has a devastating effect on their mental health.

Nursing studies also have identified significant strengths in battered women, indications of normal processes of grieving and recovering, and cultural and social support influences on responses to battering (e.g., Hoff, 1990; Landenburger, 1989). Campbell and her colleagues demonstrated that the majority of battered women in one community sample left relationships or managed to end the violence (Campbell, Miller, Cardwell, & Belknap, 1994). Campbell (Campbell, in press; Stuart & Campbell, 1989) has also conducted research related to homicides of women in battering relationships, suggesting that nurses need to assess abused women for risk of homicide and suicide. Campbell's research, which includes a danger assessment instrument, has been

An Overview of Violence 11

partially validated by independent nursing research (Foster, Veale, & Foge, 1989).

Nursing research also has begun to consider the children of battered women. These children are at risk for health, school, and emotional problems, as well as increased aggressiveness, which may continue into adult violence (Humphreys, 1993). Humphreys (1990, 1991) has investigated how abused women and their children care for each other, in spite of the dangers of their situation. Using qualitative methodology, Ericksen and Henderson (1992) documented the powerlessness, uncertainty, and sadness of these children and their needs for nursing intervention. Henderson (1989) found that children's responses to abusive situations greatly influenced their mother's decision making.

Elder Abuse

Two programs of nursing research on elder abuse have been particularly influential. Phillips and Rempusheski (1986) documented the difficult decision making of nurses to determine the best course of action to take for abused elders. Phillips (1983) also tested a model of elder abuse that emphasized providing support for caregivers of the elderly. Fulmer and colleagues (Fulmer & Ashley, 1989; Fulmer, Street, & Carr, 1984) have developed and tested an Elder Abuse Assessment instrument that now has substantive reliability and validity. They have also identified the risk factors of functional disability, confusion, minority status, and poor social networks for elder maltreatment, with cognitive impairment more associated with neglect than with abuse (Fulmer, McMahon, Baer-Hines, & Forget, 1992; Lachs, Berkman, Fulmer, & Horowitz, 1994).

Child Abuse

Building on Burgess' pioneering research on child sexual assault (Burgess, Groth, Holstrom, & Sgroi, 1978), Kelley's (1989) national study of children sexually abused in child care found increased behavior problems in comparison to matched controls. In continuing studies, Kelley (1992,1993) also reported a relationship between maternal use of illicit drugs and child maltreatment, and found that grandparents caring for formerly abused grandchildren experienced increased stress, social isolation, and role restriction. Other nursing researchers have investigated the effects of incest on women's health (Draucker, 1989; Urbancic, 1992).

Taken cumulatively, these findings indicate data-based nursing interventions that in many cases support the clinical suggestions already in the literature (e.g., Henderson, 1989; King & Ryan, 1989, Limandri, 1986). Some of the studies have small samples and/or unsophisticated methodologies; however, the findings from those studies generally support the findings of more advanced research, both inside and outside nursing (see Campbell & Parker, 1992, for a more complete and critical review of nursing research related to battered women and their children). Most exciting in this research is the emphasis on strengths, rather than pathology, the inclusion of cultural issues, and the implications for interventions that empower victims of violence rather than patronize them.

UNIQUE PERSPECTIVE OF NURSING RESEARCH

An advocacy orientation is apparent in nursing research on family violence. Nursing studies have avoided much of the victim blaming and emphasis on pathology characteristic of other disciplines' research that has viewed women victimized by violence as a deviant group (Campbell, 1991; Schur, 1980; Wardell, Gillespie, & Leffler, 1983). In addition, nurse researchers have intervened with those victimized by violence, either by working directly with the women or by providing staff training. Nurses also have made clinical suggestions in research reports. These nursing contributions often go beyond what has been found in studies and reflect nurses' concerns and rich clinical backgrounds. These additions are not usually guided by a theoretical or philosophical premise of emancipation, but reflect the clinical grounding of nursing research and the recognition of survivors' needs for empowerment. For example, the findings from one nursing study (Campbell & Alford, 1989) influenced one state to no longer exempt marital rape from prosecution.

Nursing research on victimization has approximated a critical theory approach (Allen, 1986). Those victimized by violence are most often members of disenfranchised groups, of minority ethnic groups, and/or women or children. Research has shown that health care professionals contribute to the further subjugation of these people. For instance, health professionals are more likely to report poor and minority parents for child abuse than middle-class white couples whose children have comparable injuries (Newburger, Newburger, & Hampton, 1983). Health care professionals also are more likely to derogatorily label, tranquilize, and give inappropriate care to battered women in the emergency department than to other patients (Kurz, 1987; Stark, Flitcraft, & Frazier, 1979). One reason that these professionals may try to distance themselves from victims of violence and the problem of violence is the perception that it is a problem of an "other" or deviant group. It is encouraging to have research demonstrate that at least in one area of violence, wife abuse, practicing nurses are less likely than physicians to blame victims for the violence directed against them (Rose & Saunders, 1986). The majority of nurses in another sample, however, did *not* routinely screen for family violence and intervene with the victims of this violence (Tilden et al., 1994).

It is also important that nursing research has begun to explore cultural issues related to violence (e.g., McFarlane et al., 1992; Rodriguez, 1993; Torres, 1987), and that most studies have been ethnically heterogeneous. Nurse researchers have used a variety of philosophical and methodological approaches to study violence, including both qualitative and quantitative analysis of data. By supporting the validity of similar findings from contrasting methodologies, nursing research has enriched the knowledge base about violence.

Nursing research has generally grown out of clinical concerns rather than a deductive, theoretical testing approach. Thus, nursing research is generally congruent with the calls for an "activist research agenda" proposed by those who align themselves with the grassroots sexual assault and battered women's movement, Afrocentric theory, feminist theory, and critical theory (Dobash & Dobash, 1988). These researchers and activists want to ensure that the primary agenda for future research empowers the men, women, and child victims (rather than blaming them) and places the responsibility to change on the social system rather than on the individual (Lee & Harris, 1993). Nurse researchers' knowledge of and ability to influence the health care system, combined with their social consciousness and clinical concerns, gives them a unique and crucial part in this agenda.

PREVENTION APPROACHES

Healthy People 2000 has identified the reduction of injuries due to violence as a major public health goal for the United States. Surveillance systems, the necessary foundation for studying any public health problem, are needed to help define the extent of this problem. The next step in the public health approach to violence-related injuries is to conduct research to identify risk factors and develop and test interventions. Nurses should participate in all facets of this injury research, but it is especially important that they help collect data on injuries and contribute to the design of surveillance systems. Nurses must also implement interventions to reduce violence and injuries from violence, and measure their effectiveness.

Haddon has proposed a matrix model of injury prevention strategies that can be applied to violence-related injuries (Haddon, 1980). Haddon's matrix consists of three distinct phases of the injury (pre-event, event, and post-event) on the left hand side, and the target of the intervention (host, agent, and environment) across the top. Haddon (1980) suggests that strategies be planned for all boxes in the matrix. He also outlines 10 useful prevention strategies, which are listed in Table 1.1. Nurses participating in injury research can use these strategies to design successful prevention programs.

POLICY IMPLICATIONS

The nursing discipline is poised to make a substantive contribution to local, state, and national policy on violence. The American Academy of Nursing (AAN) has recognized this policy opportunity by appointing an Expert Panel on Violence and devoting its 1993 annual conference to the topic. The AAN and the American Nurses Association (ANA) have contributed to national violence prevention and reduction efforts in all branches of government (ANA, 1980; Campbell et al., 1993), along with specialty nursing organizations such as the Emergency Nursing Association and the Association of Women's Health, Obstetric, and Neonatal Nurses (AWHONN, formerly NAACOG). The nursing discipline has contributed data and policy recommendations to the

TABLE 1.1. Haddon's 10 Injury Prevention Strategies

1. Prevent the creation of the hazard (stop producing poisons; stop manufacturing guns).
2. Reduce the amount of the hazard (package toxic drugs in smaller, safe amounts; manufacture less lethal bullets).
3. Prevent the release of a hazard that already exists (make bathtubs less slippery; raise drinking age laws).
4. Modify the rate or spatial distribution of the hazard (require automobile air bags; make and enforce gun registration laws.)
5. Separate, in time and space, the hazard from that which is to be protected (use sidewalks to separate pedestrians from automobiles; lock up unloaded guns).
6. Separate the hazard from that which is to be protected by a material barrier (insulate electrical cords; wear bicycle helmets).
7. Modify relevant basic qualities of the hazard (make crib slat spacings too narrow to strangle a child; require trigger locks on all guns).
8. Strengthen the resistance of the victim (teach conflict resolution strategies; gun safety education).
9. Begin to counter the damage already done by the hazard (provide emergency medical care).
10. Stabilize, repair, and rehabilitate the object of the damage (provide acute-care and rehabilitation facilities; license suspension/revocation for drunk drivers).

An Overview of Violence 15

ongoing program of violence prevention of the Centers for Disease Control's Intentional Injury Division, and nursing has offered policy suggestions for achieving the 18 violence reduction objectives of *Healthy People 2000* (Campbell et al., 1993).

The Nursing Network on Violence Against Women International (NNVAWI), formed in 1985, has formulated policies on violence and advocated for increased information on violence in nursing curricula and inservice programs. This effort has included the collection and dissemination of information on courses, protocols, and training materials available through regular NNVAWI conferences and in the NNVAWI column in the journal *Violence Update.* NNVAWI supports the current bill before the House of Representatives, chiefly sponsored by Oregon Representative Wyden, which mandates the inclusion of information on domestic violence in the basic curricula of all health care professionals. NNVAWI members have worked with the National Coalition on Domestic Violence and state coalitions, local shelters, state and local health departments, and many schools of nursing. They have presented at regional and national conferences, including American Nurses Association (ANA), National League for Nursing (NLN), NAACOG, and Sigma Theta Tau International. What is still needed from these and other national nursing organizations is more systematic national activity through coordination, directives, bulletins, and board-level action.

Also needed is increased coordination between nursing and national organizations, such as the Black Women's Health Network and the National Women's Health Network, on issues of violence that affect women. These coalitions can advocate for more stable funding for abuse care and for the expansion of wife-abuse shelters throughout the country. Such development can help bring to fruition the United States Department of Health and Human Services (USDHHS, 1990) objective to reduce to less than 10% (from 40% currently) the proportion of battered women turned away from shelters for lack of space.

A similar coordinated effort between nursing and pertinent consumer health organizations can address the separate year 2000 objectives to increase the number of identified child abuse victims receiving appropriate care and to extend protocols for identifying all assault and abuse victims to 90% of emergency departments. Thanks in part to the efforts of NNVAWI, the National Coalition Against Domestic Violence, and especially the Pennsylvania Coalition Against Domestic Violence, the 1992 Joint Commission on the Accreditation of Hospitals Organization (JCAHO) standards included a stipulation for just such protocols in emergency departments, alcohol abuse treatment centers, and ambulatory care centers. The 1994 JCAHO standards widen this mandate to *all* inpatient and outpatient health care facilities accredited by the organization. Nurses should work with the state coalitions against domestic violence and with emergency departments to ensure that those new protocols include feasible, legitimate, and appropriate outlines for abuse identification and nursing interventions. Systematic coordination on this issue is also needed at the national level, among the ANA, the Emergency Nurses Association, the NNVAWI, gerontological organizations, and other appropriate groups.

Other nursing efforts to prevent violence are needed in schools. Conflict resolution programs have been implemented throughout the country, and school nurses need to be part of the team implementing these efforts. Such education needs to include gender-specific conflict resolution information and discussion, so that issues of power and control in male–female relationships, date rape, other forms of dating violence, and attitudes toward women are added to the more common gender neutral or male-male forms of conflict resolution curriculum materials. The Community Health practice council of ANA, the National Association of School Nurses, the Public Health Nursing Section of the American Public Health Association (APHA), and the U.S. Public Health Service can be the nucleus of a working coalition to advocate and shape such curricula. The National Coalition Against Domestic Violence has date violence curriculum materials that can be used to further these efforts.

Coalitions of maternal–child nursing organizations, interdisciplinary child abuse associations, and the Children's Defense Fund are needed to prevent child abuse. These coalitions can draw attention to violence prevention by advocating parental education programs, such as the proper storage of firearms in the home. Nurses should also be an integral part of existing interdisciplinary hospital child abuse and neglect "teams." These teams were organized in almost all hospitals in the 1970s, but have lost impetus in many hospitals in the last decade.

The overwhelming majority of homicides, suicides, and injuries from assault are caused by handguns. The financial costs of guns to our nation in terms of emergency care, intensive care, spinal cord injury rehabilitation, surgery, stoma care, and general medical care have yet to be accurately tabulated. Nursing needs to participate in the many initiatives around the country working toward decreasing this devastation from guns. While additional analytic studies are needed, especially studies of nonfatal firearm injuries, present studies suggest that the protective effects of gun ownership should be questioned.

Existing programs of nursing research, nursing organizations, and individual nurses have changed national policy on the prevention of violence and abuse so that the health care system is now a major contributor to the solution of this national horror. With systematic, coordinated efforts and leadership from within nursing, this foundation can become even more influential. Nursing must continue to be in the forefront of developing scholarship on violence and using that knowledge to provide leadership for change in health care policy. By continuing to emphasize the early identification of victims of

An Overview of Violence   17

violence and providing interventions that decrease the numbers of repeat
victims or perpetrators, nursing can change the quality of life in this country
and improve the health of its citizens.

REFERENCES

Allen, R. B. (1986). Measuring the severity of physical injury among assault and
    homicide victims. *Journal of Quantitative Criminology, 2*, 139-156.
American Nurses Association. (1980). *Nursing: A social policy statement.* Kansas
    City, MO: American Nurses Association.
Baker, S., O'Neill, B., Ginsburg, M., & Guohua, L. (Eds.). (1992). *Injury fact book.*
    New York: Oxford University Press.
Block, M. R., & Sinnott, J. D. (1979). *Battered elder syndrome: An exploratory study.*
    College Park: University of Maryland, Center on Aging.
Brendtro, M., & Bowker, H. L. (1989). Battered women: How can nurses help? *Issues
    in Mental Health Nursing, 10*, 169-180.
Bristowe, E., & Collins, J. B. (1989). Family mediated abuse of noninstitutionalized
    frail elderly men and women living in British Columbia. *Journal of Elder Abuse
    and Neglect, 1*, 45-64.
Bullock, L., & McFarlane, J. (1989). Higher prevalence of low birthweight infants born
    to battered women. *American Journal of Nursing, 89*, 1153-1155.
Bullock, L., McFarlane, J., Bateman, L. H., & Miller, V. (1989). The prevalence and
    characteristics of battered women in a primary care setting. *Nurse Practitioner,
    14*, 47-55.
Bureau of Justice Statistics. (1992). *Criminal victimization in the United States, 1990.*
    Washington, DC: U.S. Government Printing Office.
Burgess, A., Groth, A., Holmstrom, L., & Sgroi, S. (1978). *Sexual assault of children
    and adolescents.* Lexington, MA: D.C. Heath.
Burgess, A. W., & Holmstrom, L. L. (1974). Rape trauma syndrome. *American Journal
    of Psychiatry, 131*, 981-986.
Burgess, R. I., & Draper, P. (1989). The explanation of family violence: The role of
    biological, behavioral, and cultural selection. In L. Ohlin & M. Tonry (Eds.),
    Family violence (pp. 59-116). Chicago: University of Chicago Press.
Campbell, J. C. (1989a). A test of two explanatory models of women's responses to
    battering. *Nursing Research, 38*, 18-24.
Campbell, J. C. (1989b). Women's responses to sexual abuse in intimate relationships.
    Women's Health Care International, 8, 335-347.
Campbell, J. C. (1991). Public health conceptions of family abuse. In D. Knudson &
    J. Miller (Eds.), *Abused and battered* (pp. 35-48). New York: Aldine de Gruyter.
Campbell, J. C. (in press). Prediction of homicide of and by battered women. In
    J. Campbell (Ed.), *Assessing the risk of dangerousness: Potential for further
    violence of sexual offenders, batterers, and child abusers,* Newbury Park,
    CA: Sage.
Campbell, J. C., & Alford, P. (1989). The dark side of marital rape on women's health.
    American Journal of Nursing, 89, 946 949.
Campbell, J. C., Anderson, E., Fulmer, T. L., Girouard, S., McElmurry, B., & Raff, B.
    (1993). AAN working paper: Violence as a nursing priority: Policy implications.
    Nursing Outlook, 41(2), 83-92.

18   *Nursing Care in a Violent Society: Issues and Research*

Campbell, J., & Fishwick, N. (1993). Abuse of female partners. In J. Campbell & J. Humphreys (Eds.), *Nursing care of survivors of family violence* (pp. 68-104). St. Louis: Mosby.

Campbell, J. C., Miller, P., Cardwell, M. M., & Belknap, R. A. (1994). Relationship status of battered women over time. *Journal of Family Violence, 9*, 99-111.

Campbell, J. C., & Parker, B. (1992). Battered women and their children. In J. J. Fitzpatrick, R. L. Taunton, & A. K. Jacox (Eds.), *Annual Review of Nursing Research* (Vol. 10, pp.77-94). New York: Springer Publishing Company.

Campbell, J. C., Pliska, M. J., Taylor, W., & Sheridan, D. (in press). Battered women's experiences in emergency departments: Need for appropriate policy and procedures. *Journal of Emergency Nursing.*

Campbell, J. C., Poland, M. L., Waller, J. B., & Ager, J. (1992). Correlates of battering during pregnancy. *Research in Nursing and Health, 15*(3), 219-226.

Campbell, J., Smith-McKenna, L., Torres, S., Sheridan, D., & Landenburger, K. (1993). Nursing care of abused women. In J. Campbell & J. Humphreys (Eds.), *Nursing care of survivors of family violence* (pp. 248-289). St. Louis: Mosby.

Centers for Disease Control. (1992). Homicide surveillance - United States, 1979-1988. *MMWR, 41*(SS-3), 1-34.

Cicirelli, V. (1983). Adult children's attachment and helping behavior to elderly parents: A path model. *Journal of Marriage and the Family, 45*, 815-825.

Daro, D. (1988). *Confronting child abuse: Research for effective program design.* New York: FreePress.

Dobash, R. E., & Dobash, R. (1988). Research as social action: The struggle for battered women. In K. Yllo & M. Bograd (Eds.), *Feminist perspectives on wife abuse* (pp. 51-74). Beverly Hills, CA: Sage.

Draucker, C. B. (1989). Cognitive adaptation of female incest survivors. *Journal of Consulting and Clinical Psychology, 57*(5), 668-670.

Ericksen, J. R., & Henderson, A. D. (1992). Witnessing family violence: The children's experience. *Journal of Advanced Nursing, 17*, 1200-1209.

Federal Bureau of Investigation. (1991). *Uniform crime reports for the United States, 1990.* Washington, DC: U.S. Government Printing Office.

Fingerhut, L. A., & Kleinman, J. C. (1989). Firearm mortality among children and youth. *Advance data from vital and health statistics of the Centers for Disease Control, No. 178.* Hyattsville, MD: National Center for Health Statistics.

Foster, L. A., Veale, C. M., & Foge, C. I. (1989). Factors present when battered women kill. *Issues in Mental Health Nursing, 10*, 273-284.

Fulmer, T., & Ashley, J. (1989). Clinical indicators of elder neglect. *Applied Nursing Research, 2*, 161-167.

Fulmer, T., McMahon, D., Baer-Hines, M., & Forget, B. (1992). Abuse, neglect, abandonment, violence and exploitation: An analysis of all elderly patients seen in one emergency department during a six-month period. *Journal of Emergency Nursing, 18*(6), 505-510.

Fulmer, T., Street, S., & Carr, K. (1984) Elder abuse screening and detection in the emergency unit. *Journal of Emergency Nursing, 10*, 131-140.

Gelles, R. J. (1974). Child abuse as psychopathology: A sociological critique and reformulation. In S. Steinmetz & M. Straus (Eds.), *Violence in the family* (pp. 190-204). New York: Dodd, Mead.

Gil, D. G. (1970). *Violence against children: Physical child abuse in the United States.* Cambridge: Harvard University Press.

Gin, N., Rucker, L., Frayne, S., Cygan, R., & Hubbell, A. (1991). Prevalence of domestic violence among patients in three ambulatory care internal medicine clinics. *Journal of General Internal Medicine, 6*, 317-322.

An Overview of Violence   19

Goldberg, W. G., & Tomlanovich, M. C. (1984). Domestic violence victims in the emergency department. *Journal of the American Medical Association, 251*, 3259-3264.

Gondolf, E. W., & Foster, R. A. (1991). Wife assault among VA alcohol rehabilitation patients. *Hospital and Community Psychiatry, 42*, 74-79.

Haddon, W. (1980). Advances in the epidemiology of injuries as a basis for public policy. *Public Health Reports, 95*, 411-421.

Hamberger, L. K., Saunders, D. G., & Hovey, M. (1992). Prevalence of domestic violence in community practice and rate of physician inquiry. *Family Medicine, 24*, 283-287.

Hampton, R. L., & Newberger, E. H. (1985). Hospitals as gatekeepers: Recognition and reporting in the national incidence study of child abuse and neglect. *Report to the National Center on Child Abuse and Neglect.* Washington, DC: Children's Bureau, Office for Human Development Services, U.S. Department of Health and Human Services.

Helton, A. S., McFarlane, J., & Anderson, E. T. (1987). Battered and pregnant: A prevalence study. *American Journal of Public Health, 77*, 1337-1339.

Henderson, A. D. (1989). Use of social support in a transition house for abused women. *Health Care for Women International, 10*, 61-73.

Hoff, L. A. (1990). *Battered women as survivors.* London: Routledge.

Humphreys, J. C. (1990). Dependent care of battered women and their children. *MAINlines, 11*(1), 6-7.

Humphreys, J. C. (1991). The children of battered women: Worries about their mothers. *Pediatric Nursing, 17*, 342-345.

Humphreys, J. C. (1993). Children of battered women. In J. Campbell & J. Humphreys (Eds.), *Nursing care of survivors of family violence* (pp.. 107-131). St. Louis: Mosby.

Kalmuss, D. (1984). The intergenerational transmission of marital aggression. *Journal of Marriage and the Family, 47*, 11-19.

Kellermann, A. L., & Mercy, J. A. (1992). Men, women, and murder: Gender-specific differences in rates of fatal violence and victimization. *Journal of Trauma, 33*, 1-5.

Kellermann, A. L., & Reay, D. T. (1986). Protection or peril? An analysis of firearm-related deaths in the home. *New England Journal of Medicine, 314*, 1557-1560.

Kellermann, A. L., Rivara, F. P., Rushforth, N. B., Banton, J. G., Reay, D. T., Francisco, J. T., Locci, A. B., Prodzinski, J., Hackman, B. B., & Somes, G. (1993). Gun ownership as a risk factor for homocide in the home. *New England Journal of Medicine, 329*, 1084-1091.

Kelley, S. J. (1989). Stress responses of children to sexual abuse and ritualistic abuse in day care centers. *Journal of Interpersonal Violence, 4*, 502-513.

Kelley, S. J. (1992). Parenting stress and child maltreatment in drug-exposed children. *Child Abuse and Neglect: The International Journal, 16*, 317-328.

Kelley, S. J. (1993). Caregiver stress in grandparents raising grandchildren. *Image: Journal of Nursing Scholarship, 25*, 331-337.

Kempe, C. H., Silverman, F. N., Steele, B. F., Droegemueller, W., & Silver, H. K. (1962). The battered child syndrome. *Journal of the American Medical Association, 181*, 17-24.

King, M. C., & Ryan, J. (1989). Abused women: Dispelling myths and encouraging intervention. *Nurse Practitioner, 14*, 47-58

Klaus, J. F. (1987). Homicide while at work: Persons, industries, and occupations at high risk. *American Journal of Public Health, 77*, 1285-1289.

Kurz, D. (1987). Emergency deparment responses to battered women: Resistance to medicalization. *Social Problems, 34*, 501-513.

Lachs, M. S., Berkman L., Fulmer T., & Horwitz, R. I. (1994). A prospective community-based pilot study of risk factors for the investigation of elder mistreatment. *Journal of the American Geriatrics Society, 42*(2), 169-173.

Landenburger, K. (1989). A process of entrapment in and recovery from an abusive relationship. *Issues in Mental Health Nursing, 10*, 209-227.

Lee, R. K., & Harris, M. J. (1993). Unintentional firearm injuries: The price of protection. *American Journal of Preventive Medicine, 9*(Suppl. 1), 16-20.

Lee, R. K., Waxweiller, R. J., Dobbins, J.G., & Paschetag, T. (1991). Incidence rates of firearm injuries in Galveston, Texas, 1979-1981. *American Journal of Epidemiology, 134*, 511-521.

Limandri, B. J. (1986). Research and practice with abused women: Use of the Roy adaptation model as an explanatory framework. *Advances in Nursing Science, 8*, 52-61.

McFarlane, J., Parker, B., Soeken, K., & Bullock, L. (1992). Assessing for abuse during pregnancy: Severity and frequency of injuries and associated entry into prenatal care. *Journal of the American Medical Association, 267*, 3176-3178.

Moore, M. H. (1993). Violence prevention: Criminal justice or public health? *Health Affairs, 12*(4), 34-45.

National Center for Health Statistics. (1993). *1991 U.S. compressed mortality data* [Public use data tape]. Washington, DC: Centers for Disease Control.

National Research Council. (1993a). *Understanding child abuse and neglect.* Washington, DC: National Academy Press.

National Research Council. (1993b). *Understanding and preventing violence.* A. J. Reiss, Jr. & J. A. Roth (Eds.). Washington, DC: National Academy Press.

Newberger, E. H., Newberger, C. M., & Hampton, R. L. (1983). Child abuse: The current theory base and future research needs. *Journal of the American Academy of Child Psychiatry, 22*, 262-268.

Okun, L. (1986). *Woman abuse: Facts replacing myths.* Albany, NY: State University of New York.

Olds, D. L., & Kitzman, H. (1990). Can home visitation improve the health of women and children at environmental risk? *Pediatrics, 86*(1), 108-116.

Parker, B., & McFarlane J. (1991). Feminist theory and nursing: An empowerment model for research. *Advances in Nursing Science, 13*, 59-67.

Parker, B., McFarlane, J., & Soeken, K. (1993). Abuse of pregnant adolescents. *Nursing Research, 42*, 173-178.

Phillips, L. R. (1983). Abuse and neglect of the frail elderly at home: An exploration of theoretical relationships. *Journal of Advanced Nursing, 8*, 379-392.

Phillips, L. R., & Rempusheski, V. F. (1986). Making decisions about elder abuse. *Social Caseworker, 67*, 131-140.

Pillemer, K., & Finkelhor, D. (1988). The prevalence of elder abuse: A random sample survey. *Gerontologist, 28*(1), 51-57.

Pillemer, K., & Frankel, S. (1991). Domestic violence against the elderly. In M. L. Rosenberg & M. A. Fenley (Eds.), *Violence in America: A public health approach* (pp. 158-183). New York: Oxford University Press.

Rodriquez, R. (1993). Violence in transience: Nursing care of battered migrant women. *AWHONN's Clinical Issues in Perinatal and Women's Health Nursing, 4*(3), 437-440.

Rose, K., & Saunders, D. G. (1986). Nurses' and physicians' attitudes about women abuse: The effects of gender and professional role. *Health Care for Women International, 7*, 427-438.

Schur, M. E. (1980). *The politics of deviance: Stigma contests and the uses of power.* Englewood Cliffs, NJ: Prentice Hall.

An Overview of Violence 21

Sengstock, M. C., & Liang, J. (1983). Domestic abuse of the aged: Assessing some dimensions of the problem. In *Interdisciplinary topics in gerontology (Vol. 17). Social gerontology.* New York: S. Karger.

Shalala, D. (1994, May/June). Domestic abuse epidemic in the U.S. *The Nation's Health,* p. 6.

Shiferaw, B. S., Mittlemark, M. B., Wofford, J. L., Anderson, R. T., Walls, P., & Rohrer, B. (1994). The investigation and outcome of reported cases of elder abuse: The Forsyth County Aging Study. *Gerontologist, 34*(1), 123-125.

Sniezek, J. E., Finklia, J. F., & Graitcek, P. L. (1989). Injury coding and hospital discharge data. *Journal of the American Medical Association, 262,* 2270-2272.

Sorenson, S., & Peterson, J. (1994). Traumatic child death and documented maltreatment history, Los Angeles. *American Journal of Public Health, 84,* 623-627.

Stark, E., & Flitcraft, A. H. (1991). Spouse abuse. In M. Rosenberg & M. Fenley (Eds.), *Violence in America: A public health approach* (pp. 123-157). New York: Oxford University Press.

Stark, E., Flitcraft, A., & Frazier, W. (1979). Medicine and patriarchal violence: The social construction of a "private" event. *International Journal of Health Services, 9*(3), 461-493.

Steinmetz, S. K. (1978). The battered husband syndrome. *Victimology, 2,* 499-502.

Straus, M. A., & Gelles, R. J. (1986). Societal change and change in family violence from 1975 to 1985 as revealed by two national surveys. *Journal of Marriage and the Family, 48,* 465-479.

Straus, M. A., Gelles, R. J., & Steinmetz, S. K. (1980). *Behind closed doors: Violence in the American family.* New York: Doubleday.

Stuart, E. P., & Campbell, J. C. (1989). Assessment of patterns of dangerousness with battered women. *Issues in Mental Health Nursing, 10,* 245-260.

Tilden, V. P., Schmidt, T. A., Limandri, B. J., Chiodo, G., Garland, M. J., & Loveless, P. (1994). Factors that influence clinicians' assessment and management of family violence. *American Journal of Public Health, 84,* 628-633.

Tilden, V. P., & Shepherd, P. (1987). Increasing the rate of identification of battered women in an emergency department: Use of a nursing protocol. *Research in Nursing and Health, 10,* 209-215.

Torres, S. (1987). Hispanic-American battered women: Why consider cultural differences? *Response, 10*(3), 20-21.

Trimpey, M. L. (1989). Self-esteem and anxiety: Key issues in an abused women's support group. *Issues in Mental Health Nursing, 10,* 297-308.

Ulrich, Y. C. (1991). Women's reasons for leaving abusive spouses. *Health Care for Women International, 12,* 465-473.

Urbancic, J. C. (1992). Empowerment support of adult female survivors of childhood incest. *Archives in Psychiatric Nursing, 6,* 275-281.

U.S. Department of Health and Human Services. (1981). *Study methodology: National study of the incidence and severity of child abuse and neglect* (DHHS Publication No. OHDS 81-30326). Washington, DC: U.S. Government Printing Office.

U.S. Department of Health and Human Services. (1988). *Study findings: Study of the national incidence and prevalence of child abuse and neglect* (Contract No. 105-85-1702). Washington, DC: U.S. Department of Health and Human Services.

U.S. Department of Health and Human Services, Public Health Service (1990). *Healthy people 2000; National health promotion and disease prevention objectives.* Washington, DC: U.S. Government Printing Office.

U.S. Department of Justice. (1993). *Crime in the United States - 1992: Uniform crime reports.* Washington, DC: Federal Bureau of Investigation.

22   *Nursing Care in a Violent Society: Issues and Research*

U.S. Department of Justice. (1994). *Criminal victimization in the United States -1992: National crime victimization survey report* (Publication No. NCJ-145125). Washington, DC: Bureau of Justice Statistics.

U.S. Senate, Special Committee on Aging. (1983). *Developments in aging: 1983.* Washington, DC: U.S. Government Printing Office.

Utech, M. R., & Garrett, R. R. (1992). Elder and child abuse: Conceptual and perceptual parallels. *Journal of Interpersonal Violence, 7*(3), 418-428.

Waller, A., Baker, S., & Szocka, A. (1989). Childhood injury deaths: National analysis and geographic variations. *American Journal of Public Health, 79,* 310-315.

Wardell, L., Gillespie, D. L., & Leffler, A. (1983). Science and violence against wives. In R. Gelles, G. Hotaling, M. Straus, & D. Finkelhor (Eds.), *The dark side of families* (pp. 69-84). Beverly Hills: Sage.

Weingourt, R. (1990). Wife rape in a sample of psychiatric patients. *Image: Journal of Nursing Scholarship, 22,* 144-147.

Wolf, R. S. (1994). Elder abuse: A family tragedy. *Aging International, 21*(1), 60-64.

2

Battered Women's Anxiety for
Their Children: A Study

Janice Humphreys

Battered women's worries about their children have been reported as signifi-cantly influencing their own behaviors, including the decision to leave abusive relationships. The purpose of this study was to describe battered women's worries about their children and their responses to those worries. An ethnog-raphy using the method described by Spradley (1979) was conducted. Quali-tative analysis of the data revealed two themes about battered women's worries about their children and their responses to those worries. While the abusive adult male was a source of worry, violence outside the home was pervasive and hazardous to children. Battered women's experiences reflect the work of worrying; that is, the constant and energy-depleting nature of this difficult and vitally important process.

"At school there's a lot of fighting and drugs. My oldest daughter, she seen her Dad fighting with me a lot. She doesn't start fights, but anyone messes with her, she'll kick their butt."

Battered women have many worries. Among the most important are their worries about their children. Battered women's worries about their children have been reported as significantly influencing their own behaviors, including the decision to leave abusive relationships (Torres, 1991; Ulrich, 1991). Yet, the nature of battered women's worries about their children and their responses is largely unknown. A significant source of battered women's worries is violence in their households. Children's responses to the battering of their mothers have been well documented (Humphreys, 1994). One might assume that battered women do not worry about anything but battering. Clinical experience with battered women and their children in women's shelters and elsewhere, however, suggests that other sources of worry within their larger environment also are perceived to be threatening to their children. Therefore, the purposes of this study were to describe battered women's worries about their children and their responses to those worries.

24   *Nursing Care in a Violent Society: Issues and Research*

REVIEW OF THE LITERATURE

Mothers' Worries

Despite lengthy discussions in popular child-rearing texts and frequent references in anecdotal reports, little research has been directed toward mothers' worries about their children after the postpartum and neonatal periods. Mothers' worries and related anticipatory guidance during the first year of life have received considerable attention by nurse-researchers (Adams, 1963; Bull, 1981; Gruis, 1977; Pridham, 1993; Sumner & Fritsch, 1977).

Research on mothers' worries at later times in their children's lives has addressed maternal concerns at preventive child health visits (Wasserman, Inui, Barriatua, Carter, & Lippincott, 1983) and reasons for seeking urgent pediatric treatment (Feigelman et al.,1990; Turk, Litt, Salovey, & Walker, 1985). These reports and others (Lurie, 1974) surveyed mothers' worries in order to analyze interactions with the formal medical care system. Feigelman and associates (1990) noted that for urban families enrolled in a primary health care program, parents'—most often mothers'—worries about their children were the most significant indicator for seeking health care in the emergency room. Unfortunately, the content of those worries was not reported.

Other research has surveyed the relationship between socioeconomic status and parents' cognitive/affective responses to nuclear war (Hamilton, Knox, & Keilin, 1986). Still other reports, while presenting descriptions, focused upon the overconcern of one mother (Banks, 1977) or mothers' worries as predictors of child psychopathology (Schaefer, Hunter, & Edgerton, 1987). While the importance of mothers' worries about their children has long been recognized (Meadow, 1969), the nature of those worries has yet to be described in depth.

Battered Women

Nursing research has advanced knowledge about mothers' and children's responses to family violence (Campbell & Parker, 1992). Others have noted that mothers' responses to family violence have been reported as influencing the magnitude of the effect of violence upon their children (Jaffe, Wolfe, & Wilson, 1990; Wolfe, Jaffe, Wilson, & Zak, 1985). While violent conflict occurs all too frequently in families (Finkelhor, Gelles, Hotaling, & Straus, 1983), there is little to describe the worries and responses of mothers on behalf of their children.

Preliminary research (Humphreys, 1989) acknowledged the importance of battered women's worries about their children. In Humphreys' research, battered women's worries about their children could be categorized according to the following general patterns: the effect of violence and aggression on their children; the quality of children's home (physical) and school (academic)

Battered Women and Their Children

environments; children's personal development; and substance abuse. The focus of this research, however, was primarily battered women's dependent-care actions on behalf of their children. Identification of mothers' worries was only peripherally addressed. Nevertheless, Humphreys noted that many of the sources of worry had nothing to do with the violence and aggression at home. Rather, multiple sources of violence (at school, in the community, at home) and other causes for worry were reported. Richer detail and description of this intriguing phenomenon was deemed necessary for the purpose of sensitization (Knafl & Howard, 1984).

Worry, Anxiety and Obsession

Worry as a concept is familiar to everyone. Within the professional literature, worry has only recently received empirical study. In much of the literature worry is used interchangeably with anxiety, a situation that is now being recognized (Bruhn, 1990; McCann, Stewin, & Short, 1991). Most researchers address the phenomenon of worry, as it serves as a key component to the DSM-III-R criteria for Generalized Anxiety Disorder (American Psychiatric Association, 1987). Thus, much of the research that addresses worry does so with clinical populations in order to distinguish the role of worry separate from anxiety. Others (Freeston et al., 1994; Tallis & Silva, 1992) seek to discriminate between obsession and worry as both relate to another anxiety disorder, Obsessive-Compulsive Disorder, also as defined in the DSM-III-R. There is agreement in the literature that the distinguishing criteria of worry, anxiety, and obsession are unclear. Where distinctions are made, however, the following general characteristics of each are suggested.

Worry or apprehensive expectation is common to everyone. Bruhn (1990) proposes that worry is a process wherein individuals, through mental activity, gain information and learn new ways of dealing with potentially detrimental circumstances. Worrying is problem solving and can allow for the rehearsal of anticipated events. Bruhn suggests that worry is a way of experiencing distress without being overwhelmed by it.

Anxiety is conceptualized as an emotional reaction to an unknown, intangible, subjective, unconscious danger. In contrast, an emotional reaction to known, tangible, objective, and conscious sources of danger is defined as fear (Bruhn, 1990). McCann, Stewin, and Short (1991) envision anxiety as physiological activity in response to arousal, and worry as the cognitive process.

Obsession has commonalities with worry as well. In research with both clinic and nonclinic populations, obsession and worry were present and the content was not significantly different for either group (Turner, Beidel, & Stanley, 1992). Turner and associates, in distinguishing between worry and obsession noted the following differences: Worry is characterized as largely

26 *Nursing Care in a Violent Society: Issues and Research*

self-initiated in response to specific internal or external events, common to circumstances of everyday living. Obsession involves uncontrollable thoughts, images, and impulses that are considered unacceptable to the individual, lead to subjective distress, and often are accompanied by some form of resistance (Rachman, 1985). Worries prompt action (Turner, Beidel, & Stanley, 1992). Obsession prevents productive problem solving and often results in compulsive behaviors that, while reducing anxiety in some cases, consume the individual's time and energy.

The focus of the study reported here was battered women's worries. No effort was made to define the concept of worry for the women. In fact, the purpose of the research was to learn the intrinsic character and content of battered women's worries about their children and their responses to those worries. It is through the examination of the lives of battered women and their children that the body of knowledge is expanded and greater clarity may be provided on both their experience and the phenomenon of interest in its many manifestations.

METHOD

Sample

A purposive sample of 25 women residing at a battered women's shelter in southeastern Michigan participated in the study. The shelter was located in an area serving urban, suburban, and rural women. Twenty women were interviewed once and five women were interviewed twice. Repeat interviews with previous informants, though rare due to the short-term nature of most women's stay at the shelter (30 days), allowed for validation and extension of the data analysis. Interviews varied in length from 1 to 2 hours. None of the women informed about the research refused to participate.

Women ranged in age from 17 to 60 years ($M = 28.4$). Eleven (44%) were African American and 14 (56%) were European American. All women in the study had at least one child and one woman had 10 children ($M = 2.4$). Fifty-nine percent of the children where female and 41% were male. By their report, battered women over the previous year experienced several episodes of physical violence of varying severity at the hands of their abusive male partners. There was marked variability in the time the women reported as having been in a violent adult relationship. It ranged from less than a year to 10 years ($M = 4.3$, $SD = 2.3$, $Md = 3$). Slightly more than one third (36%) reported a history of violence between their parents. All the women in the study were admitted to the shelter because at that time they were battered, or feared that they were going to be battered, by their adult male partners. During the course of interviews, one woman described an incident which might be defined

Battered Women and Their Children   27

as child abuse by her partner; however, no other evidence of battering of children was identified by intake workers or researchers. None of the women had been in the shelter for 30 days prior to this admission and policy prevented their remaining in the shelter longer than 30 days.

Design

Data were collected through ethnographic interview and participant observation by the principal investigator (PI) and research associate (RA). A growing body of literature has advocated for the qualitative approach as the method of choice in descriptive research, especially in those areas where subjective experiences are essential for understanding (Hall & Stevens, 1991). Spradley (1979) explains that ethnography allows the researcher "to see alternative realities and modify our culture-bound theories of human behavior" (p. 13). This was thought particularly appropriate, given that others have advocated for the "need to work very hard to find strengths in the women we treat and to work through our own frustration and reactivity to bizarre and difficult behaviors of battered women, which do indeed make sense from another frame of reference" (Bograd, 1988, p. 481). Thus, an ethnography using the qualitative method outlined by Spradley (1979) was conducted.

Women were interviewed, following the pattern described by Spradley (1979), for the purpose of answering the following research questions: (1) What worries do battered women have about their children? and (2) What are the responses of battered women to worries about their children?

Data Collection Procedures

All data were collected with consideration to the rights of human subjects and followed the protocol advocated by Parker and Ulrich (1990). To further assure the safety of the shelter women, and at the request of the staff, interviews were not tape recorded. Instead detailed written records of ethnographic interviews were kept by the PI and RA within 24 hours of interviews, with particular attention to accuracy. Data were transcribed into the microcomputer by the PI and reviewed by the interviewer (PI or RA) for accuracy within days of each interview. The PI and RA met routinely to discuss the data collection and analysis process. Data analysis was facilitated through the use of NUDIST, a qualitative data analysis software.

Data Analysis

Data were analyzed following the Developmental Research Sequence described by Spradley (1979,1980). No attempt was made to compartmentalize the data according to source of worry. For example, worries resulting from violence in the home were not separated out from other sources of violence. Rather, commonalities across data were used to guide data analysis, regardless of source. The data analysis process began with the wide focus of battered women's worries about their children and their responses, and narrowed as domain and components were realized. Data were analyzed to develop descriptive questions, analyzed further to reveal domains of the phenomena, validated via structural questions, and organized into taxonomies for further analysis. Themes of battered women's worries and responses were the intended outcome of this process. For example, the investigators began with the broadest possible descriptive question: "What kinds of worries do you have about your children?" Effort was made to use the informants' own words in order to obtain their world view of the phenomenon of concern. "Some mothers have told me there are worries or every day worries or fears. Is that something you would say? How would you say it?"

After in-depth interviews with multiple informants, domain analysis was conducted to identify semantic relationships inherent in the data. For example, "Not knowing what our new home gonna be like" was identified by an informant as a reason to worry. Thus, another instance of "reason to worry" was noted. All the data collected up until that time were analyzed to find like examples, like relationships, and like domains. Structural questions were then developed to further clarify each example, relationship, and domain. An example of a structural question might be "Do you worry about some of your children differently from the others?" Or, "In what ways does your experience make your worries different from other mothers?" Each step in the process of interviewing, analyzing, validating, and interviewing led to greater clarity and specificity. Most informant interviews combined several of the steps in the analysis process. For example, a battered woman might be asked to list worries she has about her children, give her opinion about other women's worries, differentiate types of worries, and elaborate on reasons for different types of worries about her children.

Card sorting and sentence completion techniques were used throughout the data collection phase. For example, an informant might be given a stack of cards, each bearing one kind of worry described by an informant. This informant would be asked to sort the cards into piles that represented different kinds of worries to her. Upon conclusion of this process, the interviewer and informant would proceed through each stack and the informant would explain what was unique about that stack of cards and why she included each card in the stack. The process of data collection and analysis was repeated and modified with each informant based upon the obtained results and the outcome of efforts to enhance the credibility, transferability, dependability, and confirmability of the study findings.

Credibility, transferability, dependability, and confirmability were addressed according to Lincoln and Guba's (1985) guidelines. These terms refer

Battered Women and Their Children

to the degree to which qualitative research findings can be trusted as accurate reflections of informants' perspectives. Specific techniques used to enhance the trustworthiness of the research findings are identified in Table 2.1. All were incorporated within the study.

Ethnographic interviewing and participant observation techniques were employed throughout the study. While the PI and RA primarily came to the shelter to conduct interviews, during the time spent in the battered women's shelters they both observed and participated in any activities in progress. For example, the time immediately following the evening meal was often a good one for interviewing women. Upon arrival at the shelter the meal might still be in progress or after-meal-clean-up under way. Both the PI and RA immediately helped in serving or cleaning, if appropriate, and frequently brought cookies for dessert. All interactions within the environment of the shelter were noted and documented, even if not directly related to an interview. Results reflect themes derived from all sources of data.

TABLE 2.1. Techniques Used to Establish Credibility, Transferability, Dependability, and Conformability

Credibility
    Learning the context
        Extensive background and experience
          -in area of family violence
          -with mothers and children
    Reflexive journal
        Daily log, methods log, personal log
    Triangulation
        Two researchers and close monitoring of intrateam communication
    Peer debriefing
    Member checks
        1. At each interview
        2. Critique of case studies by
          -battered women
          -shelter staff
          -experts
Transferability
    Thick description
        Detailed information obtained about informant group
Dependability and Confirmability
    Research audit
        Investigation process, data analysis, interpretations, & conclusions
        reviewed by outside expert

RESULTS

Qualitative analysis of the data revealed two themes about battered women's worries about their children and their responses to those worries. They are: (1) keeping your children safe, and (2) creating order out of disorder. These themes reflect the work of worrying, that is, the constant and energy-depleting nature of this difficult and vitally important process. It is via the work of worrying that battered women attempt to protect their children and create a positive environment within the severe constraints of their lives. While the specific circumstances of a worry might vary by a child's gender or ethnic group, these themes remained constant across all battered women. Prior to a discussion of the specific themes, general findings about battered women's worries about their children are presented.

Battered women report worries about their children and violence. Sources of violence are common, however, and often *unrelated* to the abusive adult males in their lives. Sources of violence included schools (e.g., peers, guns, gangs) and the community at large (e.g., neighbors, drug dealers, police raids, robberies, strangers). Violence, as manifested in sexual abuse, is a worry even in the selection and retention of child care. Violence within the lives of battered women and their children is so pervasive as to cross boundaries into all areas of their lives. For battered women, violence outside the home was a significant source of worry about their children.

Battered women report variety in the intensity and type of worries they experience about their children. To indicate these differences, battered women refer to "worries" or "everyday worries" and "fears." The intrinsic characteristics of worries and fears vary in several ways, including intensity. "Fears are the number one worry." They also vary in their likelihood of happening and in the degree of severity of outcome. As one informant stated:

> Worries are more likely to happen, or if they happen they are not too serious or they are things that cross my mind, but probably won't happen. Fears are terrible. If she was in a car accident, she could be killed. The really awful stuff that might happen, those are my fears. Worries are more trivial than fears, but they're not trivial.

Even worries, though less intense than fears, take a physical and mental toll on battered women. Informants reported an array of physical and psychological symptoms as a result of both worries and fears. Even if an informant identified only worries about her child, she might still report experiencing a lot of physical and mental distress.

Not all battered women have the same worries about their children. Every mother, however, voluntarily voiced worries and/or fears about child care. Reasons for different worries were based upon characteristics of the child, experiences of the mother, or circumstances of both the child and the mother. Child characteristics that resulted in different worries were the child's gender,

Battered Women and Their Children 31

gestation, birth order, age, and health. Mothers felt strongly that their past life experiences resulted in different worries about their children. "Only another person with the same experiences could have the same worries about their own children." Finally, the particular circumstances of both mothers and children resulted in different worries. The nature of those circumstances influenced the types of worries battered women had about their children.

Keeping Your Children Safe

The first theme was _keeping your children safe_. Battered women spent an enormous amount of time and energy attempting to protect their children from threats to their well-being. The sources of these threats were found both in everyday life and in the unique characteristics of their situations and/or their children. Threats to their children frequently had nothing to do with the abusive adult male in their lives. For example, one mother voiced a concern that is common to many mothers, battered or not. "Any time they go off in a car, you know, I worry about there being a car wreck. Even if the person who's driving is careful, sometimes it's not even their fault." Another worry found in everyday life was voluntarily identified by every mother, that is, worries and/or fears about child care. "My major worry is when I go to work, about child care. You read in the newspaper so much, especially sexual abuse. Thinking about it I get a lump in my throat."

Other threats to their children were unique to their life circumstances and yet, still did not involve violence by their male abusers. Many women identified hazards to their children found in the environment in which they lived. For the women in this study, the immediate environment was the battered women's shelter:

> Especially around here. These stairs don't have gates. She is at the age when she can get into (everything) — light sockets, she goes up stairs.

For the majority of the women, their children's environment prior to admission to the shelter was impoverished and violent. Drugs were a common element either in the home, school, or community at large. Sources of violence often came from outside as well as inside the family. Violence from the adult male partner in the household was feared; however, violence also was a common worry in the neighborhood and in the schools.

> Drugs, cops running through the neighborhood, shooting going on in the neighborhood. . .I worry about AIDS and what AIDS has to do with drugs and with putting kids at risk. I'm tired of going out and picking up needles in the neighborhood.

Several women worried that their children were in danger of being kidnapped, a fear that was supported by the story of this young mother.

> I don't know where my children are. My assailant and unfortunately that's my husband, is hiding them. I did get one chance to talk to each of them for about 30

32   *Nursing Care in a Violent Society: Issues and Research*

seconds each. He's got them and he keeps moving them around so I don't know where they are. . . .When I did get to see the kids, before he'd open the door he took down all the pictures of them that were in the house . . .I found one in my wallet. That's all I have.

Other women worried about hazards associated with the characteristics of the children. For one mother, worries stemmed from the mature stature and appearance of her son.

Tony never quite fitted in. He was always big for his age. I have to remind myself that he's still just 14. Even though he says he's a man. "I'm not a boy . . .I'm not a child. I'm a man." Everyone has always expected more from him 'cause he's so big and looks older than he is.

Other mothers identified worries about their children's safety due to their race. Three different mothers gave examples:

Prejudice exists for Black men both in the world and in the court system against Black men. He (Jeffrey Dahmer) practically got off Scot free. They should have electrocuted him for what he did. If he had been a young Black man you believe that he wouldn't have gotten off so easy? If you do something that is not all that bad and you're a Black man and you get to the court system, the system treats you different. There's bias that puts you at a disadvantage...Injustice System.

I worry about my son especially, being Black and all. I want my child to know that the easy way is not always the right way. If somebody give him a $1,000 for taking a package from one place to another, he might look at that and say "my Mama could sure use that money" and think that would be an easy way of getting money. He sees that kind of thing all the time where we live.

I'm worried about the Rodney King situation. I need to raise my children. What about the father who was sent to prison when the one child shot the other? [Father was held responsible for not keeping the gun safely.] Would that happen if they were White?

Responses. Battered women described a variety of responses that were used to keep their children safe. These included vigilance and intuition, teaching their children, adjusting their own lives, having a plan, and if need be, putting themselves between danger and their children. Each of these is briefly illustrated.

Vigilance and Intuition. In the attempt to keep their children safe, women employed constant vigilance, combined with astute understanding of their children. Because much of the worry about their children was due to sources outside their family, battered women were forced to be vigilant about everything. Throughout the study, battered women referred to the need to watch their children and other people to determine the nature of a situation and, if need be, their response. One mother said, "I figure it's like there are guardian angels that look out for them (children). I believe in guardian angels. . . (But) my kids don't need a guardian angel. They have me."

Battered Women and Their Children   33

This notion of constant vigilance was time-consuming and both reassuring and exhausting. Mothers reported significant fears about not being with their children. When their children where not under their watchful eyes, battered women were even more worried and frequently initiated responses to ascertain the condition of their children. At times, it was by watching out for their children that these battered women felt reassured.

Concurrent with constant vigilance was the battered women's astute awareness of the unique characteristics of their children. Battered women analyzed situations, considered the characteristics of their children, and made judgments about the presence of current and future problems for their children. This almost instantaneous and ongoing process was fundamental to battered women's determination about worries and responses.

Continuous observation and intuition were used by battered women to monitor their children, determine if their children were in jeopardy, and to judge others for their worthiness to serve as a replacements for the women themselves.

> ...you can tell if it is okay to leave your child with somebody. There's a way they act, a way they behave either with their own child or with yours, that you get a feeling from them. Also you see how they behave. It's both observing them as well as a feeling.

The extreme difficulty of determining the worthiness of others to care for their children was voluntarily mentioned by every informant. Battered women reported that this was a heavy burden upon them that demanded the use of all their faculties. Even if a child care provider initially seemed responsible, women continued to monitor the provider's behavior and worthiness, a tiresome and never ending task critical to the safety of their children.

Teaching. Battered women used several methods to teach their children in order to protect them and keep them safe. They might serve as a role model for their child. One woman responded, "by coming here. I showed them that they don't have to be abused. That they don't have to just take it. That they always have the option to leave." They might attempt to educate their child about a perceived threat.

> I tell my 20-year-old about bump and run scams. I tell her to drive to the nearest police station. I tell her to check the battery in the smoke detector. I tell her when she goes dancing to go to the bathroom with other girls (to protect herself from an attack as a single female in the bathroom).

Or, they might attempt to establish limits to the child's behavior by using discipline and/or setting boundaries. "My boys were raised on the straight and narrow. If you look suspicious and are a Black male, you go to jail."

Adjusting Their Own Lives. Certain threats to their children's safety might be best addressed by changes in the women's own patterns of living. "She is in a difficult age, too old for a baby sitter and too young to be alone. I've tried to

34   *Nursing Care in a Violent Society: Issues and Research*

adjust my life so she won't need a baby sitter." This adjustment of work and other responsibilities can itself present a complex system of arrangements for women who, for all practical purposes, are single parents. The burden of child-rearing and supporting their families often falls completely to battered women.

Under a different threat to the safety of their children, battered women may decide to adjust their own lives by leaving an abusive relationship (Ulrich, 1991). Other research has described battered women protecting their children by removing them on a regular or permanent basis (Humphreys, in press).

Having a Plan. Women remarked upon the need to have a plan to protect their children. The plan might address the immediate situation, the future for themselves and their children, or both. "I'm going to nursing school so that I can get a job and we can have a future." For some, the plan was known only to the woman. For others, the plan was known by all. "We always have a plan with him [husband]. We all know it. If he starts drinking, we leave. If we see beer cans or if he starts acting like he's been drinking, we leave."

Putting Themselves Between Danger and Their Children. When all else fails and/or when an emergency situation requires it, mothers reported putting themselves between danger and their children. In this study, the source of danger was often the abusive adult male in the household.

> If he hadn't been drinking, he'd have passed it off and said "put the belt away." But instead he said "Didn't you hear your Mother? Take that off and put it away." And that's how it all got started. He grabbed Ted (son) by the shirt [Joyce gets up to reenact the scene for me] and pushed him against the wall and pulled his hand up into a fist. I jumped up and said "Don't you hit him." He had his hand around his neck and I put myself up between him and said "Leave him alone." So he grabs me and I said to Melody (daughter) "Call the police" and that's how we got here.

Obviously, some women put themselves in great jeopardy for the sake of their children.

Creating Order Out of Disorder

The second theme was creating order out of disorder. Battered women and their children frequently live their lives in worlds of chaos and disorder. Sources of this disorder are their life circumstances, a severe lack of resources, and at times, the mothers' and/or children's own behaviors. A significant factor contributing to the disorder in their lives is the abusive adult male. In fact, the direct threat of violence was the precipitating factor in the battered women's flight with their children to the shelter. The chaos resulting from the abusive partners, however, was only one source of disruption in their lives. Within lives of disorder, battered women sought to give purpose, reason, and order to their lives and the lives of their children. These women frequently described the tremendous responsibility they felt to create a meaningful life for their

Battered Women and Their Children   35

children. In fact, some women identified that the work to be done in the shelter was to put their lives into some kind of order.

> When you are here, it is time to reassess your life. The decisions I make affect her [daughter's] life. I want to use the time to my advantage. I come here and I have nowhere to be. I have short-term, mid-, and long-term goals. I'm thankful for the shelter—where would you go?

Battered women's shelters helped them to create order and for that they spoke with appreciation for the existence of the shelter and their advocates on staff. Their time prior to admission to the shelter and much of their lives during the time of residence, however, were fraught with tremendous turmoil.

The majority of women reported an extraordinary lack of resources to help them care for their children. Sometimes this deficit was so severe that the women feared they would have difficulty meeting even the most basic needs of their children. One of the women said, "I worry about trying to make it a life, trying to raise them by myself. I worry about how we gonna manage." For most women, future housing was an unknown. Many women were not employed, and for those who were employed, the history of battering and/or the flight to the shelter, often was associated with difficulties in maintaining employment.

> I called into the business office of the management company I work for and they've moved me to another site 36 miles away and now instead of being a manager, I'm a leasing agent (a significantly reduced position). At first they said I got mileage to and from the site and now they say I don't. He's still got the job (the one they originally shared) and the apartment and I've got nothing. I've got the certificate in a management training course and I'm the one who gets the shaft.

It was not unusual for women who were employed to report losing their jobs as a result of their flight to the battered women's shelter. With little or no income, with a sense that the decisions they make in the shelter have lifelong consequences for themselves and their children, women struggled to organize their worlds from the turmoil and disorder of the past.

Finally, women acknowledged that, at times, their children's behavior and/ or more often their own, limited the degree to which they could get themselves organized.

> Bob [son] started getting aggressive with me at home, verbally aggressive. I could see how mad he'd get. It would just come out and he'd explode. He'd get so angry. He started getting aggressive, even in school.

For this mother, her child's behavior proved a further disruption in their situation. For other mothers, this time of disorder in their own thinking and functioning as a mother seemed short-term but was of concern.

Responses. The consensus from the mothers in this study was that the most important and effective response to their worries and fears about their children

36   *Nursing Care in a Violent Society: Issues and Research*

during this chaotic time was to "let your children know that you love them."
Women attempted to freely give and show love to their children through
different methods. Women described the need to invest time in their children.

> My mother was extremely fastidious. I'm not like that. I say "let's bake a pie and
> there may be flour everywhere. But, don't worry. We can clean it up together
> later." I'm not prim and proper. I want them to have a good time.

Women reported that they accepted their children and demonstrated that
acceptance as a way to show love.

> I appreciate them for who they are. I appreciate them for what they are. My one
> daughter wants to grow up to be a mermaid. I tell her that's just fine. They don't
> have to hide or feel ashamed. I was made to feel that way. I love them enough
> to want them to be who they're going to be.

Finally, women in the study insisted that love and affection must be shown
regularly to children.

> You have to show love. You have to hug them even if they don't want to. Like
> my oldest son. He doesn't want to hug me when his friends are around. You just
> have to go up and red face and kiss them. You have to kiss them in private. You
> have to tickle them and have pillow fights.

Other ways that mothers sought to help their children through the disorder
of their lives was to help them when they needed it and talk with them about
all that was going on.

> Communicating with them. Telling them that I'm never too busy to come and
> talk to them. Teaching them to express themselves. Now they come to me
> anytime and they tell me everything. Even their friends come over and tell me
> things. They know that I tell them the truth, that I talk to them, that I listen to
> them.

Finally, women sought help for themselves as a means of helping their
children. The source of help might be the shelter personnel. A belief in God and
the ability to call for help through prayer was also a source of help to women.
"I just figure that there's a higher power. Those times when you need help, if
anyone can help, the Lord can. And to tell you the truth, in the past it's worked."

DISCUSSION

Battered women have described the work of worrying about their children and
the responses they use to take care of their children. Women have related their
dedication to protect and nurture their children against extraordinary odds. The
nature of worry by battered women in this research is consistent with much of
the reported literature. Worry was described as a mental process wherein
battered women identified potentially hazardous situations for their children
and sought to deal with them. Their worries were in response to potentially
detrimental circumstances for their children. Battered women frequently

Battered Women and Their Children

attempted to anticipate dangerous life circumstances for their children, a finding noted in Humphreys' (in press) preliminary work. Worry for battered women also was self-initiated and revolved around circumstances of everyday life for their children. For the battered women in this study, however, everyday life included worries common to all mothers (i.e., child care) as well as those common to their situation (i.e., bigotry, violence, abuse).

The lives of battered women and their children were permeated with violence. Violence directed toward the women by their male partners was a worry to all informants. Other sources of violence outside the household, however, were equally pervasive. Children of battered women were exposed to violence as they walk or ride the bus to school, in their contacts with peers, on the playground, in the streets, in the neighborhoods, and by strangers, friends, and relatives alike. Drugs, guns, and sexual abuse are a threat anywhere. Even law enforcement threatens violence for young people, especially Black males, if they are in the wrong place at the wrong time.

Battered women worry about the affects of abuse in their homes; however, they also fear for their children when they go off to school or merely to a playground. It is no wonder they reported the need to be constantly vigilant. Violence surrounds and envelops them. It is startling to hear battered women's stories about the kicks and slaps at home, but it is exhausting to hear about the multitude of dangers in the outside world. The threats to their children are everywhere, the dangers almost unlimited.

Nursing interventions directed toward diminishing the extent of violence in the lives of battered women and their children are aimed at all levels of prevention. The violence experienced by battered women and their children is reflective of the violence in the United States. The cultural tolerance for violence in the media and in our homes is shocking. While some advocate for more jails in which to house offenders, the more hopeful and powerful solution rests with each individual. Violence can only exist in a society where it is allowed and condoned by the majority of people. While no one person can stop the violence by him- or herself, we can by our actions stop its spread. Campbell and Humphreys (1994) have addressed at length the primary prevention of violence. Interventions must be directed toward diminishing the cultural tolerance for violence in every form. Interventions at the societal level require social and support services for marginal persons, public education on nonviolent conflict resolution, and educational assistance to youth at risk of becoming school drop-outs. Even small gestures, such as a refusal to buy violent, racist, and sexist toys as gifts, can decrease even the implication of approval to children and parents alike. Other obvious interventions require every nurse in every setting to assess for family violence. Nursing care that directly addresses family violence offers help to those who might otherwise go unaided and educates nonviolent families to the fact that nurses are a potential source of help, should problems occur. Violence is complex and not easily stopped. Additional study including intervention research is clearly needed.

38   *Nursing Care in a Violent Society: Issues and Research*

It is obvious that the battered women in this study had extremely limited resources. Many sources of worry reflect battered women's lack of even basic needs (i.e., money, food, shelter, employment). In fact, a primary reason for coming to the women's shelter was that they had nowhere else to go. Battered women in this research often were marginal people. Whether the worries described here are common to all marginal people is unknown. Speculation about similarities with other persons, however, must consider the significant disadvantage experienced by battered women, given their history of violence by their intimate male partners. For example, landlords are frequently hesitant to rent to battered women as they "don't want to get involved in domestic disputes." Others view battered women as unreliable especially because they may return to the abusive relationship. Furthermore, battered women, like all women, are subject to discriminatory practices in a workplace that pays women less than men for the same work. The experiences of being battered and being a woman make life within the larger environment dangerous and difficult. Further research is needed to explore the life experiences of other disenfranchised groups.

Battering of women has been defined as deliberate and repeated physical aggression or sexual assault inflicted on a woman by a man with whom she has or has had an intimate relationship (Campbell, 1989). Battering is a pattern, not a single incident. While the physical and psychological toll of battering on women has been documented (Campbell, 1989), the labor of worrying about their children has not previously been described. The demanding, exhausting, and, at times, dangerous nature of battered women's worries and responses required considerable energy and effort by the women. It is likely that this energy expenditure has limited their abilities to attend to other areas of their lives and may affect their physical and mental well-being. The degree to which the work of worrying about their children influenced women's responses to battering is unknown. In this research, however, worrying about their children was found to contribute to battered women's difficulties.

The findings of this study, that women expend considerable energy worrying about their children, suggest that the work of worrying may influence women's responses to battering and thus, the effect of violence upon their children. Research reports have noted that women's responses to battering influence the magnitude of the effect of violence upon their children (Jaffe, Wolfe, & Wilson, 1990; Wolfe, Jaffe, Wilson, & Zak, 1985). These findings and conclusions suggest that nurses who work with battered women and their children help both battered women and indirectly their children when they ease the work of worrying. These conclusions require further research and suggest implications for nursing practice. For example, nurses who provide care to battered women and their children should encourage discussion of worries. Salmon (1993) advocates that clients in stressful circumstances may benefit most by discussing their own thinking and responses. He encourages involve-

Battered Women and Their Children

ment rather than "passive" relaxation techniques for those who experience worry (moderate to high anxiety). Battered women should be told that by helping themselves, they are helping their children. This may free battered women to focus upon themselves and not feel that they are at the same time neglecting their children. Questioning should include reference to "worries" and "fears," as these terms have different meanings to battered women. Open discussion of worries and fears will, in both private and peer group settings, enable women to share their common experiences, learn and critique responses, and be reassured that they are not alone in their work.

Nurses and others associated with shelters provide hope and help to battered women and their children, within an environment of danger, and little help. Women flee to shelters with their children because they fear for their own lives and seek to improve the lives of their children. The women in this research tell of terrible worries about their children and their use of themselves as protectors and shields. They say that love given often and freely can make a difference in the lives of their children. Yet, they also tell of their constant vigilance and fear. Professionals in shelters need to make every effort to provide additional resources to overburdened women and reassure mothers and praise their efforts to protect and nurture their children. Battered women need help with basic necessities, finding safe homes, obtaining employment, or returning to school. Shelter personnel are often expert in helping women navigate social service systems to obtain food stamps, and in providing other aid. Nurses can support the process and provide health care and related services to mothers and children. For example, identification and evaluation of child-care providers can be aided through resources at state and community levels. Professionals may wish to distribute relevant brochures and share positive child-care-provider information. While in battered women's shelters, women should be encouraged to take time to organize and clarify their thoughts and plans. In turn, professionals can build upon the problem solving that the women have already done, thus enhancing their own sense of self and their accomplishments. Acknowledgment of the arduous and difficult tasks of worrying in a world wrought with violence may provide battered women with renewed energy to prevail in their responsibilities.

REFERENCES

Adams, M. (1963). Early concerns of primigravida mothers regarding infant care activities. *Nursing Research, 12*, 72-77.

American Psychiatric Association. (1987), *Diagnostic and statistical manual of mental disorders* (3rd ed., rev.). Washington, DC: American Psychiatric Association.

Banks, M. J. (1977). A family's over-concern about a child in the first two years of life. *Maternal-Child Nursing Journal, 6*(3), 187-194.

40   *Nursing Care in a Violent Society: Issues and Research*

Bograd, M. (1988). Case conference: Consultant's response. *Journal of Interpersonal Violence, 3,* 478-482.

Bruhn, J. G. (1990). The two sides of worry. *Southern Medical Journal, 83,* 557-562.

Bull, M. J. (1981). Change in concerns of first-time mothers after one week at home. *Journal of Obstetrical, Gynecological and Neonatal Nursing, 10,* 391-394.

Campbell, J. C. (1989). A test of two explanatory models of women's responses to battering. *Nursing Research, 38,* 18-24.

Campbell, J. C., & Humphreys, J. (1994). *Nursing care of survivors of family violence.* St. Louis: Mosby.

Campbell, J. C., & Parker, B. (1992). Battered women and their children. In J. J. Fitzpatrick, R. L. Tunten, A. K. Jacox (Eds.), *Annual review of nursing research,* (Vol. 10, pp. 77–94). New York: Springer Publishing Company.

Feigelman, S., Duggan, A. K., Bazell, C. M., Baumgardner, R. A., Mellits, E. D., & DeAngelis, C. (1990). Correlates of emergency room utilization in the first year of life. *Clinical Pediatrics, 12,* 698-705.

Finkelhor, D., Gelles, R. J., Hotaling, G. T., & Straus, M. A. (Eds.). (1983). *The dark side of families: Current family violence research.* Beverly Hills: Sage.

Freeston, M. H., Ladouceur, R., Rheaume, J., Letarte, H., Gagnon, F., & Thibodeau, N. (1994). Self-report of obsessions and worry. *Behavior Research and Therapy, 32,* 29-36.

Gruis, M. (1977). Beyond maternity: Postpartum concerns of mothers. *Maternal Child Nursing, 2,* 192-188.

Hall, J. M., & Stevens, P. E. (1991). Rigor in feminist research. *Advances in Nursing Science, 13*(3), 16-29.

Hamilton, S. B., Knox, T. A., & Keilin, W. G. (1986). Relationship between family socioeconomic status and cognitive/affective responses to the threat of nuclear war. *Psychological Reports, 58,* 247-250.

Humphreys, J. (1989). Dependent-care directed toward the prevention of hazards to life, health, and well-being in mothers and children who experience family violence. (Doctoral dissertation, Wayne State University, 1989).

Humphreys, J. (1994). Children of battered women. In J. C. Campbell & J. Humphreys (Eds.), *Nursing care of survivors of family violence* (pp. 107-131). St. Louis: Mosby.

Humphreys, J. (in press). Dependent-care by battered women: Protecting their children. *Health Care for Women International.*

Jaffe, P. G., Wolfe, D. A., & Wilson, S. K. (1990). *Children of battered women.* Newbury Park, CA: Sage.

Knafl, A. K., & Howard, M. J. (1984). Interpreting and reporting qualitative research. *Research in Nursing and in Health, 7,* 17-24.

Lincoln, Y. S., & Guba, E. G. (1985). *Naturalistic inquiry.* San Francisco: Jossey-Bass.

Lurie, O. R. (1974). Parents' attitudes toward children's problems and toward use of mental health services: Socioeconomic difference. *American Journal of Orthopsychiatry, 44,* 109-120.

McCann, S. J. H., Stewin, L. L., & Short, R. H. (1991). Sex differences, social desirability, masculinity, and the tendency to worry. *Journal of Genetic Psychology, 152,* 295-301.

Meadow, S. R. (1969). The captive mother. *Archives of Diseases of Childhood, 44,* 362-367.

Parker, B., & Ulrich, Y. (1990). A protocol of safety: Research on abuse of women. *Nursing Research, 39,* 248-250.

Battered Women and Their Children 41

Pridham, K. F. (1993). Anticipatory guidance of parents of new infants: Potential contribution of the internal working model construct. *Image: Journal of Nursing Scholarship, 25*, 49-56.

Rachman, S. J. (1985). An overview of clinical and research issues in obsessive-compulsive disorder. In M. Mavissakalian, S. M. Turner & L. Michelson (Eds.), *Obsessive-compulsive disorders: Psychological and pharmacological treatment* (pp. 1-47). New York: Plenum.

Salmon, P. (1993). The reduction of anxiety in surgical patients: An important nursing task or the medicalization of preparatory worry? *International Journal of Nursing Studies, 30*, 323-330.

Schaefer, E., Hunter, W. M., & Edgerton, M. (1987). Maternal prenatal, infancy and concurrent predictors of maternal reports of child psychopathology. *Psychiatry, 50*, 320-331.

Spradley, J. P. (1979). *The ethnographic interview*. New York: Holt, Rinehart & Winston.

Spradley, J. P. (1980). *Participant observation*. New York: Holt, Rinehart& Winston.

Sumner, G., & Fritsch, J. (1977). Postnatal parental concerns: The first six weeks of life. *Journal of Obstetrical, Gynecological and Neonatal Nursing, 6*, 27-32.

Tallis, F., & Silva, P. (1992). Worry and obsessional symptoms: A correlational analysis. *Behavior Research and Therapy, 30*, 103-105.

Torres, S. (1991). A comparison of wife abuse between two cultures: Perceptions, attitudes, nature and extent. *Issues in Mental Health Nursing, 12*, 113-131.

Turk, D. C., Litt, M. D., Salovey, P., & Walker, J. (1985). Seeking urgent pediatric treatment: Factors contributing to frequency, delay, and appropriateness. *Health Psychology, 4*, 43-59.

Turner, S. M., Beidel, D. C., & Stanley, M. A. (1992). Are obsessional thoughts and worry different cognitive phenomena? *Clinical Psychology Review, 12*, 257-270.

Ulrich, Y. (1991). Women's reasons for leaving spouse abuse. *Health Care for Women International, 12*(4), 465-473.

Wasserman, R. C., Inui, T. S., Barriatua, R. D., Carter, W. B., & Lippincott, P. (1983). Responsiveness to maternal concern in preventive child health visits: An analysis of clinician-parent interactions. *Developmental and Behavioral Pediatrics, 4*, 171-176.

Wolfe, D. A., Jaffe, P., Wilson, S.,& Zak, L. (1985). Children of battered women: The relation of child behavior to family violence and maternal stress. *Journal of Consulting and Clinical Psychology, 53*, 657-665.

3

Toward Effective Treatment of Abused Women: What Nurses Can Do

Marylou Yam

An alarming number of women seek help for abuse from the health care establishment. Yet research shows that all too often, professionals fail to identify abuse and are nontherapeutic. This chapter provides theoretical and research evidence to explore the factors that account for the less than helpful response of nurses toward wife-abuse victims. A feminist lens is used to explore strategies that can enable nurses to deal effectively with this health care dilemma.

Wife abuse is a world-wide health problem. In 1990, in its publication outlining objectives for health care, the United States Department of Health and Human Services listed violent and abusive behavior as one of the 22 priority issues of *Healthy People 2000*. In this discussion, wife abuse is defined as the use of physical force (battering) by a male toward his female partner. The term wife abuse is being used since other labels for wife abuse such as family violence or spouse abuse mask the dimensions of gender and power that are basic to an understanding of the problem (Bograd, 1988). Moreover, these terms hide the data (Hoffman, 1992; U.S. Commission on Civil Rights, 1982) that show that the majority of violence in the home is directed at female members by male members.

Statistics indicate that every year 1.5-to-2-million women seek medical help for wife-abuse injuries (Browne, 1987). In a survey of emergency department nurses employed at several hospitals in a metropolitan area ($n = 62$), respondents reported seeing a range of 1 to 60 wife-abuse victims per year with a mean of eight clients, and 52 of these nurses reported encountering a range of 1 to 15 wife-abuse victims per month with a mean of three clients (Yam, 1993).

In spite of the large numbers of women who seek help for abuse-related injuries, the evidence reveals that health care professionals neglect to uncover the etiology (McLeer & Anwar, 1989; Randall, 1990; Varvaro, Wolfinger, & Jones, 1993). In a November 6, 1991 letter to the editor of the *New York Times*, the Executive Director of the New York State Office for the Prevention of Domestic Violence, Karla Digirolamo suggested that, according to recent

43

44   *Nursing Care in a Violent Society: Issues and Research*

statistics, "25% to 40% of all injuries of women in emergency rooms are related to domestic violence. Yet health care providers may identify only 3% of these injuries as abuse related" (p. A24). Moreover, researchers have charged that nurses and other professional helpers fail to implement protocols (Kurz, 1987; Warshaw, 1989), blame victims (Flitcraft & Stark, 1989; Kurz, 1987), are unsympathetic (Drake, 1982), and do not view wife abuse as a legitimate health problem (Kurz, 1987).

By not providing effective help, health care professionals are permitting a chronic and potentially fatal problem to exist. Ultimately, nurses in practice need to be able to identify victims[1] and to provide interventions that will empower these women. The purposes of this chapter are to elucidate the factors that account for the less than effective response of health care professionals toward wife-abuse victims and to demonstrate how the discipline of nursing can more effectively help these women. An overview of the prevalence of wife abuse is followed by research findings that illustrate how the health care establishment has responded to these clients. The underlying factors that impede a therapeutic response are discussed, as are strategies that can enable nurses to effectively deal with this health care dilemma.

THE PREVALENCE OF WIFE ABUSE

Statistics reveal that 1.8 million women in the United States are battered by their male partner each year (U.S. Department of Health and Human Services, 1991). Battering is the most common cause of injury to women, being more common than automobile accidents, muggings, and rapes combined (Stark & Flitcraft, 1988).

An abused woman's physical trauma can be acute and/or chronic. Acute trauma can range in severity from bruises to gunshot wounds. Besides acute traumatic injuries, some abused women present symptoms thought to be the result of the stress of living in a violent relationship. These chronic symptoms include frequent psychophysiological illnesses, joint pain, and/or tenderness (Campbell & Humphreys, 1993), leg pain, multiple-site pain, abdominal pain, low-back pain, and headaches (Haber & Roos, 1985).

Psychological problems such as depression, and self-destructive behaviors such as drug abuse and alcoholism, may result from the pain of being battered. It has been estimated that 30% to 50% of female psychiatric patients have a health history that includes abuse (New Jersey Department of Consumer Affairs, 1990). Furthermore, approximately 50% of all female alcoholism develops in the context of on-going abuse (Flitcraft & Stark, 1989). Battering may account for 50% of suicide attempts among black women and 25% of all

Wife Abuse 45

such attempts by non-black women (New Jersey Department of Consumer Affairs, 1990). For some women, abuse is fatal; approximately 1,000 women are beaten to death annually in the United States (American Nurses Association, 1991).

THE HEALTH PROFESSIONAL'S LACK OF RESPONSE TO WIFE-ABUSE VICTIMS

In light of these alarming statistics, effective help for this population is of paramount importance. Research evidence, however, demonstrates that the response and action of health care providers has not been therapeutic. In many instances health professionals fail to identify abuse. Warshaw (1989) reviewed the emergency room charts of 52 cases in which the woman was intentionally injured by another person. Of the 52 charts reviewed, nurses failed to record information about abuse in 15% of the cases; the physician did not report it in 21%. Varvaro, Wolfinger, and Jones (1993) reviewed 468 emergency department medical records of adult female patients who were classified as trauma cases. In 94% of the charts there was no documented cause of injury or information on the record about abuse.

Even when abuse is identified, helpers treat these women in a derogatory manner, blame them for their predicament, and do not implement protocols. Warshaw's (1989) study revealed that "there was no psychiatry consult in 96% of the 52 cases reviewed, no social work consult in 92%, and no shelter information or referral sheet given in 98% of the cases" (p. 510). Drake's (1982) study illustrated the uncaring attitude of health professionals toward wife-abuse victims. In this investigation, none of the women conveyed positive feelings about the health care received. They described instances of impersonal care, lack of support, and disinterest in their problems on the part of nurses and physicians. In a more recent study, battered women who had received care in the emergency department reported that health care providers failed to ask about abuse, belittled their dilemma and showed a lack of caring (Campbell, Pliska, Taylor, & Sheridan, 1994). Kurz (1987) studied the responses of staff members to wife-abuse victims in four hospital emergency departments. In three of the hospitals, where staff did not have ongoing training on abuse, in only 11% of cases of probable battery did staff respond positively, that is, with referral to services, thorough documentation, follow-up care, and empathic interviewing. In the fourth hospital emergency department where staff had ongoing training, 47% of the cases were rated as positive. Kurz (1987) also reported that in 40% of their encounters, staff members described wife-abuse victims as possessing deviant traits such as being "crazy" and "evasive" (p. 75).

UNDERLYING FACTORS FOR THE INEFFECTIVE RESPONSE TO WIFE-ABUSE VICTIMS

Several explanations have been documented to account for the ineffective care of wife-abuse victims by health professionals. Reasons include the helpers' use of the Medical Model approach (Burge, 1989; Flitcraft & Stark, 1989; Warshaw, 1989), nurses' and physicians' beliefs in cultural myths and stereotypes about women (Bograd, 1982; Kurz, 1987), the helpers' beliefs that wife abuse is not a legitimate problem, and the helpers' beliefs that he or she cannot do much to successfully assist the wife-abuse victim (Kurz, 1987). In addition, King (1988) and Yam (1993) found that educators fail to address content on wife abuse in nursing curricula. Thus, many nurses lack the knowledge required to identify and help wife-abuse victims.

The Medical Model is one where the focus of help is on the presenting of physical ailments, not their underlying cause. Furthermore, the Medical Model promotes passivity rather than action on the part of the client. The use of the Medical Model for helping abused women has received much criticism, since it prevents the helper from attending to the etiology of wife abuse (Burge, 1989; Warshaw, 1989). Burge (1989) pointed out that the "health problems surrounding victimization tend to get neglected because the etiology falls outside the realm of biological systems and thus doesn't 'fit in' the medical education system" (p. 372). Given this explanation, it seems that in using the Medical Model approach, health professionals restrict their help to treatment of the woman's medical problems but do not address the abuse. Data exist to support this claim. In the previously mentioned Warshaw (1989) study, in more than 90% of the 52 cases, the physician did not obtain a psychosocial history, did not ask about sexual abuse or a past history of abuse, did not ask about the woman's living arrangements, and failed to ask about the woman's safety. These findings indicate that in many instances the symptoms resulting from the abuse are addressed, but the primary problem, the battering, is ignored.

Research evidence reveals that nurses, too, endorse a medical approach in their interventions with abused women. Yam (1993) examined the models of helping among emergency department nurses in relation to wife-abuse victims. The Models of Helping and Coping, proposed by Brickman et al. (1982), was the framework used to operationalize the kind of help the nurse endorsed. Brickman and others (1982) explicated four models of helping and coping that describe what form a person's behavior will take in a helping relationship. The four models of helping are: Enlightenment Model, Moral Model, Medical Model, and Compensatory Model. Each model delineates the view of the client, the role of the helper, and the form of help to be given. Brickman and others (1982) explained that one's endorsement of a particular model of help

Wife Abuse

is based on one's decision about who is responsible for the cause of, and solution to the client's problem.

According to Brickman and others (1982), the Medical Model is one where the client is viewed as weak or ill. In this model, clients are not held responsible for the cause of the problem, and the helper is responsible for solving the problem. The form of help to be rendered is a type of treatment or material aid. Clients are expected to be compliant with the prescribed regimen. The model is not empowering, in that the person to be helped assumes a passive, dependent role and the helper serves as rescuer.

Of the 106 emergency department nurses sampled, Yam (1993) found that almost half of the nurses, or 49% (n = 52), preferred a Medical Model approach in helping wife-abuse victims. In another study, using the Models of Helping and Coping, King (1988) reported that among 53 emergency department nurses, 74% (n = 39) endorsed the Medical Model of helping in their interventions with wife-abuse victims. Thus, these two studies revealed that the majority of nurses sampled preferred a model of help that fostered a dependent helper–helpee relationship.

Additionally, Yam (1993) found a significant negative correlation between the nurses' endorsement of the Medical Model and the number of victims the nurse reported seeing per year (r = -.22, $p < .05$). In other words, the less frequently the nurse endorsed the Medical Model of help, the greater the number of wife-abuse victims the nurse reported encountering per year. This finding lends support to the literature that asserts that the Medical Model of helping is to blame for the failure of health care professionals to identify wife-abuse victims.

Another reason for the ineffective care of these women is that cultural myths and stereotypes frequently deter practitioners from asking about abuse (Bograd, 1982). Some of the findings from Kurz's (1987) study supported this claim. In her investigation, for example, one nurse stated: "A lot of women do things to provoke a man. Probably most of them do. I know there are some really crazy women around here." And another nurse stated, "Well, it is normal for a woman to fight with a man in this area" (Kurz, 1987, p. 76). This researcher also reported that health professionals did not view battering as a legitimate medical concern and that staff did not believe they were able to do much to help the abused woman (Kurz, 1987).

Additionally, the less than helpful response among nurses may be due to the failure of educators to include the issue of wife abuse in nursing curricula. In Yam's (1993) study, only 34% of 106 emergency department nurses reported receiving education on the issue of wife abuse in their basic professional nursing education. In 1988, King reported that only 20% of 116 nurses claimed they had content on wife abuse in their basic program. How can nurses identify wife-abuse victims if they are not taught how to assess for victimization? How can nurses be helpful to wife-abuse victims if they are not instructed in strategies of empowerment for these women?

RECOMMENDATIONS FOR A THERAPEUTIC RESPONSE

First, in order to uncover abuse and effectively help abused women, the issue of wife abuse needs to be addressed in nursing curricula. Second, practitioners need to shift their approach of help for these women from one of rescuing to one of empowering. In other words, rather than focus on attempts to control or solve the woman's predicament, nurses must empower women to make their own choices.

Educating About Wife Abuse

Several authors (Campbell, 1992; King & Ryan, 1989; Tilden, 1989) have urged nurse educators to teach students about abuse. In 1991, the American Nurses Association released a Position Statement on Physical Violence Against Women in which it specifically recommended that health care professionals be educated in the prevention, assessment, and intervention of physical violence against women. All students must learn about this issue in basic professional programs. The discipline of nursing cannot afford to offer material on abuse solely in an optional elective course. If educators offer the content only as an elective, the issue is perceived as nonessential, and the legitimacy of abuse as a health problem is reduced. Such token courses deny some students the opportunity to learn how to identify and help wife-abuse victims.

Furthermore, increasing the opportunity for nurses already in practice to learn about abuse is critical. Yam (1993) found that 61% of 106 nurses sampled did not receive an in-service or training session on wife abuse from their institution of practice. These data support the need for health care institutions to offer such training.

Given the previously discussed research that revealed that nurses endorse a Medical Model approach for helping wife-abuse victims, that they hold negative stereotypes about these women and that they do not view wife abuse as a legitimate health issue, the goals of instruction should include:

- Having students examine their beliefs about abuse and the women who are victimized;
- Making students aware of the statistics indicating the prevalence of abuse; and
- Teaching assessment skills to identify abuse, as well as interventions and resources to empower victimized women.

These goals can best be accomplished by incorporating a personal approach to the teaching of abuse. Within the discipline of nursing, Benner (1984) found that expert nurses had first to come to terms in some personal way with what the client was confronting before they became good at working with clients with a particular problem. Feminist educators, as well, value personal experience in learning (Schniedewind, 1987). Sharing on a personal level makes content relevant to one's life and work. In order to facilitate a personal perspective, students need to hear the stories of women who have been abused. Campbell (1992) asserted that "the only way we will get students to be excited and energized and empathetic in their practice with survivors of violence is for them to get to know these women as people just like themselves" (p. 464). Survivors of intimate violence, which may include nurses, could be invited to class to share what they have undergone. Dialogue with these women can heighten students' sensitivity to the abused woman's plight, so that they are able to make sense of her fear, courage, and ability to survive.

Students who have experienced violence in their lives also need the opportunity to share their stories. Reactions to readings and course materials in the form of journal entries, logs, reaction papers, or small group discussions may provide them with an outlet for conveying their personal experiences and stimulate all students to examine their attitudes and beliefs about abuse.

Frequent exposure of students to wife-abuse victims is another important teaching element. Benner (1984) stated that in an effort to comprehend and accept the "otherness" of clients, "nurses get a head start on this understanding through personal experience of their own and through frequent experiences with patients with a particular problem" (p. 68). Yam (1993) reported that approximately 15% of the nurses sampled claimed that they learned from their clinical experience with abused women and/or their personal experience how to help wife-abuse victims. Perhaps the nurses who claimed that they came to know about wife-abuse victims through their clinical interactions with these women were in effect learning to see and to attend to cues in these clients that are reflective of abuse. Given Yam's finding and Benner's observation of the value of frequent exposure, it seems imperative that opportunities to interact with abuse victims and those who work with them are essential if practitioners are to have the skills necessary to identify and help these women.

There are numerous ways in which students can be exposed to wife-abuse victims and expert helpers. As already stated, inviting survivors of abuse to class can provide a safe place for students to become familiar with these women prior to clinical exposure. Nurses, faculty, community activists, and other professionals who have experience working with these victims can serve as individual or panel presenters and discussion leaders. These individuals enable students to learn about resources available for abused women, serve as role models for change, and provide specific information on how to help abused women. Agencies devoted to helping these women, such as battered women's shelters and community mental health centers, can be a source of

50   *Nursing Care in a Violent Society: Issues and Research*

opportunities for internships and/or clinical placements. Campbell (1992) asserted that experience with wife-abuse victims can occur in any clinical setting where nurses encounter adult women.

Action-oriented learning strategies are also beneficial in teaching about wife abuse, including such activities as reading and reflecting on articles in the popular literature, writing a letter to the editor, accessing information, and supporting legislation that addresses wife abuse. These activities enable students to view the problem of wife abuse on a personal level, view the problem in the broader political context of violence against women, and be agents of change.

The Nursing Response in Practice: Empowering Abused Women

A feminist perspective on wife abuse is used to inform an understanding of how to perceive the abused woman, clarify the nature of the nurse's role as helper, and derive strategies for interventions that enable wife-abuse victims to reclaim their lives. Feminists view patriarchal norms and society's condoning of violent behavior as major reasons for the cause and maintenance of wife abuse (Bograd, 1988; Kurz, 1989). Patriarchy is defined as the "manifestation and institutionalization of male dominance over women and children in the family and the extension of male dominance over women in society in general" (Lerner, 1986, p. 239). With regard to male domination, Bograd (1988) argued that "the reality of domination at the social level is the most crucial factor contributing to and maintaining wife abuse at the personal level" (p. 14). From a feminist perspective, wife abuse restrains women from controlling their lives. Thus, in order to help wife-abuse victims, feminists advocate strategies that are aimed at increasing the woman's self-respect and independence (Schechter, 1987). In the nursing literature, several authors, including Campbell and Sheridan (1989) and King and Ryan (1989), stress interventions aimed at empowering abused women. Specific empowering strategies include acknowledging the abuse, listening, avoiding blaming, exploring options, and making referrals. The following guidelines can assist nurses to empower wife-abuse victims.

Examine One's Attitude Regarding Wife-abuse Victims. In order to effectively help these women, the first step is to raise one's consciousness about the stereotypes concerning wife abuse and wife-abuse victims. Unless the myths are shed, such biases will interfere with the nurse's ability to be therapeutic (King & Ryan, 1989). Each nurse must examine his/her personal attitude toward abused women. Questions to heighten personal awareness of stereotypical notions may include:

Do I blame the woman for her predicament?
Do I see the abused woman as a powerless victim?
Do I think the abused woman is able to participate in freeing herself from the controlling relationship?

Wife Abuse   51

Bograd (1984) stressed that feminist values are clear on the attribution of responsibility for blame in wife-beating incidents: for example, "(1) no woman deserves to be beaten; (2) men are solely responsible for their actions" (p. 561). Schechter (1987) echoed this sentiment, claiming that helpers must convey to the woman that she is not responsible for the abuse. Approaches that blame the woman for her predicament can reinforce a feeling of powerlessness.

View the Abused Woman as an Able Participant in the Helping Relationship. In order to empower an abused woman, the nurse needs to view the woman as an individual who can make decisions and collaborate with others to solve her dilemma. Bograd (1988) claimed that in contrast to the more prevalent view of battered women as helpless victims or as provocative women, feminists approach battered women as survivors of life-threatening situations who are adaptive and have many strengths. From a feminist perspective, the role of the helper should raisie questions such as "What do you want to do?" "In what way can I be helpful to you?" (Schechter, 1987, p. 13).

Utilize Strategies that Empower. When operating from a Medical Model, health professionals believe that it is their role to be in control of the questions and to solve the client's problem. Abused women often present with symptoms that do not fit neatly into a preexisting medical category (Burge, 1989). Cues may be ignored or considered irrelevant by the nurse and, consequently, many women go undetected.

When helpers shed the Medical Model approach, they provide abused women with an opportunity to speak about the factors surrounding their physical conditions. These women cannot be hurried. They need time to ventilate their feelings to a helper who is nonjudgmental and empathic.

Routinely, all women involved in an intimate relationship with a man should be asked questions to uncover abuse (Campbell & Humphreys, 1993; Tilden, 1989). The literature indicates that it is not uncommon for victims to deny abuse and/or its severity (Douglas & Dionne, 1991). Women may suffer feelings of shame, embarrassment, fear, and self-blame. Guidelines for communicating with wife-abuse victims are well documented in the nursing literature (Campbell & Humphreys, 1993; King & Ryan, 1989; Noel & Yam, 1992; Tilden, 1989). Providing privacy, making eye contact, empathizing, listening, and offering options may encourage women to discuss the problem.

Authors articulating a feminist perspective have persistently urged helpers to allow women to make their own decisions (Noel & Yam, 1992; Schechter, 1987). Nurses need to work *with*, not *for*, abused women. For example, by providing information about shelters and support groups and by acknowledging the woman's strengths and courage, the helper empowers the woman to take charge of her future. Making referrals can be a challenge when the abuser is present during the health care visit. Efforts must be made to

52   *Nursing Care in a Violent Society: Issues and Research*

interview the client alone. Also, information about options can be placed in women's restrooms. These clients may be reluctant to take written materials, since their partner may inspect their belongings. In these instances, offering to make calls and telling women how and where they can locate assistance may be helpful.

Support for the use of a model of empowerment for abused women was demonstrated by Yam (1993). Of the 10 nurses who reported being victims of abuse, 50% selected a model of help that reflected empowerment. Results, using the chi-square statistic, revealed that a significantly larger proportion of nurses who were abused selected this model as compared with the total sample, $(x^2(N = 106) = 5.41, p < .02)$. This finding implies that nurses who have survived the pain of abuse may understand the need for the woman to be empowered and to take action to resolve the predicament.

SUMMARY

It is apparent from the literature that ample data exist to support the claim that health professionals have been less than helpful toward wife-abuse victims. Researchers have generated many reasons for the lack of effectual care. Because the issue of abuse is often not included in the education of nurses, there is little, if any, opportunity to counter the negative attitudes toward victims, teach students to view wife abuse as a legitimate health problem, and implement appropriate therapeutic strategies.

The means by which the discipline of nursing can develop a therapeutic response is to design curricula in nursing to take into account the issue of wife abuse and to establish training programs in all health care settings for nurses already in practice. Incorporating a personal approach to the teaching of abuse, along with frequent exposure to abused women, is stressed. Nurses need to reconceptualize their view of wife-abuse victims as strong women who can collaborate in their care, and to employ strategies to empower these women.

As indicated by the literature presented, there is a plethora of research studies describing the nontherapeutic response of helping professionals toward wife-abuse victims. Research is needed to describe effective helping between the abused woman and the nurse. Knowledge gained from exploring the essence of effective helping between the wife-abuse client and the nurse can be directed at changes in practice and suggest nursing interventions for meeting the needs of these women. In addition, more research needs to be conducted testing the effectiveness of empowerment strategies in helping wife-abuse victims.

NOTE

[1]The word victim is used to acknowledge the person who is victimized and does not intend to mean or imply that the women are powerless and/or passive.

Wife Abuse

REFERENCES

American Nurses Association. (1991). Position statement on physical violence against women. Washington, DC: American Nurses Association.

Benner, P. (1984). *From novice to expert*. Menlo Park, CA: Addison-Wesley Publishing Co.

Bograd, M. (1982). Battered women, cultural myths and clinical interventions: A feminist analysis. In New England Association for Women (Eds.), *Current feminist issues in psychotherapy* . New York: Haworth Press.

Bograd, M. (1984). Family systems approaches to wife battering: A feminist critique. *American Journal of Orthopsychiatry, 54* (4), 558-568.

Bograd, M. (1988). Feminist perspectives on wife abuse. In K. Yllö & M. Bograd (Eds.), *Feminist perspectives on wife abuse* (pp. 11-26). Newbury Park, CA: Sage Publications.

Brickman, P., Rabinowitz, V. C., Coates, D., Cohn, E., Kidder, S., & Karuza, J. (1982). Models of helping and coping. *American Psychologist, 37* (4), 368-384.

Browne, A. (1987). *When battered women kill*. New York: The Free Press.

Burge, S.K. (1989). Violence against women as a health care issue. *Family Medicine, 21* (5), 368-373.

Campbell, J., Pliska, M., Taylor, W., & Sheridan, D. (1994). Battered women's experiences in the emergency department. *Journal of Emergency Nursing, 20* (4), 280-288.

Campbell, J. (1992). Ways of teaching, learning and knowing about violence against women. *Nursing and Health Care, 13,* (9), 464-470.

Campbell, J., & Humphreys, J. (1993). *Nursing care of survivors of family violence*. St. Louis: Mosby-Year Book, Inc.

Campbell, J., & Sheridan, D. (1989). Emergency nursing interventions with battered women. *Journal of Emergency Nursing, 15*(1), 12-17.

Digirolamo, K. M. (1991, Nov. 6). Letter to the editor. *New York Times*, p. A24.

Douglas, M. D., & Dionne, D. (1991). Counseling and shelter services for battered women. In M. Steinman (Ed), *Woman battering: Policy responses* (pp. 113-130). Cincinnati, OH: Anderson Publishing.

Drake, V. (1982). Battered women: A health care problem in disguise. *Image: The Journal of Nursing Scholarship, 14* (2), 40-47.

Flitcraft, A. H., & Stark, E. (1989). Women battering: A prevention-oriented approach. In Stark, E. & Flitcraft, A. H. (Eds.), *Domestic violence: Survivors and their assailants* (pp. 56-74). New York: Garland Press.

Haber, J. D., & Roos, I. (1985). Effects of spouse abuse and/or sexual abuse in the development and maintenance of chronic pain in women. *Advances in Pain Research and Theory, 9,* 889-895.

Hoffman, J. (1992, February 16). When men hit women. *The New York Times Magazine*, p. 26.

King, M. C. (1988). *Helping battered women: A study of the relationship between nurses' education and experience and their preferred models of helping*. Doctoral Dissertation, University of Massachusetts, 1988. (University Microfilms International No. 88-13, 247).

King, M. C., & Ryan, J. (1989). Abused women: Dispelling myths and encouraging intervention. *Nurse Practitioner, 14*(5), 47-58.

Kurz, D. (1987). Emergency department responses to battered women: Resistance to medicalization. *Social Problems, 34*(1), 69-81.

Kurz, D. (1989). Social science perspectives on wife abuse: Current debates and future directions. *Gender & Society, 3*(4), 489-505.

Lerner, G. (1986). *The creation of patriarchy.* Oxford: Oxford University Press.

McLeer, S. V., & Anwar, R. (1989). A study of battered women presenting in an emergency department. *American Journal of Public Health, 79*(1), 65-66.

New Jersey Department of Consumer Affairs. (1990). *Domestic violence: A guide for health care professionals.* Trenton, NJ: Author.

Noel, N., & Yam, M. (1992). Domestic violence: The pregnant battered woman. *Nursing Clinics of North America, 27*(4), 871-884.

Randall, T. (1990). Domestic violence intervention calls for more than treating injuries. *Journal of the American Medical Association, 264*(8), 939-940.

Schechter, S. (1987). Empowering interventions with battered women. *Guidelines for mental health professionals* (pp. 9-13). Washington, DC: National Coalition Against Domestic Violence.

Schniedewind, N. (1987). Teaching feminist process. *Women's Studies Quarterly, XV* (3 & 4), 15-31.

Stark, E., & Flitcraft, A. (1988). Violence among intimates: An epidemiological review. In V. B. Van Hasselt et al. (Eds.), *Handbook of family violence* (pp. 293-318). New York: Plenum Publishing Corp.

Tilden, V. P. (1989). Response of the health care delivery system to battered women. *Issues in Mental Health Nursing, 10*, 309-320.

United States Commission on Civil Rights. (1982). *Under the rule of thumb: Battered women and the administration of justice.* Washington, DC: U.S. Government Printing Office.

United States Department of Health and Human Services. Public Health Service (1990). *Healthy People 2000: National health promotion and disease prevention objectives.* (DHHS publication number PHS 91-50212.) Washington, DC: U.S. Government Printing Office.

United States Department of Health and Human Services. (1991). *Family violence: An overview.* Washington, DC: U.S. Government Printing Office.

Varvaro, F. F., Wolfinger, K. H., & Jones, M. (1993). Documentation of abuse as cause of injury. *Violence: Nursing debates the issues* (p. 24). Maryland: American Academy of Nursing.

Warshaw, C. (1989). Limitations of the Medical Model in the care of battered women. *Gender and Society, 3*(4), 506-517.

Yam, M. (1993). *The relationship between endorsement of the compensatory model of helping and analytic style among nurses who care for wife-abuse victims in the emergency room setting.* Doctoral Dissertation, Adelphi University, 1993. (University Microfilms International No. 9416017.)

4

Preventing Child Abuse and Neglect Through Home Visitation: Hawaii's Healthy Start Program

Vicki A. Wallach and Larry Lister

Hawaii's Healthy Start program of home-based services to families identified at risk for child abuse and neglect is becoming a model for the nation. The present chapter provides background information about Healthy Start and describes a three-phase process of engagement and service delivery that characterizes the Healthy Start home visitation model.

Child maltreatment can be significantly reduced if a continuum of supportive, educational, and therapeutic services is made available to families around the time of birth (Daro, 1988). These services utilize models of practice that attend to the interrelationships among families' basic life conditions, the parents' well-being as individuals, specific aspects of parenting capacity, and healthy child development. Home visitation is increasingly regarded as a fundamental component of those programs that have been found to reduce the incidence of child abuse and neglect, and that improve the short- and long-term health and well-being of children and families.

Conclusions drawn from empirical research suggest that the provision of carefully conceptualized and implemented home visitation services does indeed reduce the incidence of child abuse and neglect (Olds, Henderson, Chamberlin, & Tatlebaum, 1986; Seitz, Rosenbaum, & Apfel, 1985). This evidence has been convincing enough that the U.S. Advisory Board on Child Abuse and Neglect, in summarizing its recommendations for dealing with the child abuse crisis in America, placed neonatal, universal home-visiting programs as a critical first step in designing a comprehensive plan to improve the overall health and safety of children (U.S. Advisory Board on Child Abuse and Neglect, 1990).

Underlying the current understanding of the importance of home visitation are theories and research findings that highlight the importance of the first years of life to the growth and development of healthy children and the value of support to their mothers who are at high risk for abuse or neglect of their children during these crucial years. The work of Winnicott (1965) on the "holding environment," of Ainsworth (1973) on "attachment," Greenspan (1981) on "reciprocity" of infant and caregiver, and Thomas and Chess (1984)

55

56   *Nursing Care in a Violent Society: Issues and Research*

on "temperament," provides some of the theoretical grounding for early intervention with mothers who may have difficulty in bonding and whose frustration
may be expressed in child abuse. Some of the research, such as the important
Kaua'i studies of child development over time (Werner & Smith, 1982) and
reports of means of reducing child abuse and neglect (Willis, Holden & Rosenberg,
1992), provides empirical support to the approaches underlying Healthy Start.
    The work of Olds and colleagues (1986) provided some of the best early
evidence that the provision of a well-defined and structured service can prevent
child abuse and neglect. In their study of home intervention with pregnant
women, which included education, enhancement of the mother's informal
support system, and linkage to community health and social services, many
positive gains were achieved. For example, among those women at greatest risk
for care-giving dysfunction, only 4% of those visited by a nurse were verified for
child maltreatment during the child's first 2 years of life, compared to 19% of
their counterparts in a comparison group.
    Given such evidence of the efficacy of early intervention approaches, there is
national debate over which components are critical for the success of home
visitation. Daro (1993), Director of Research for the National Committee to
Prevent Child Abuse and Neglect, stated: "While not all home visitation
programs are successful, those that are intensive, comprehensive, well inte-
grated into other community services and flexible in responding to a family's
unique needs produce the most consistent and impressive outcomes" (p. 4).

PURPOSE

This chapter describes one aspect of an early intervention program that is
receiving major national attention: The program is Hawaii's Healthy Start and
the component to be discussed here concerns the sequence of stages that occurs
between families and their home visitors as they work together over time.
Observations by the senior author, confirmed by other supervisors and program
directors, indicate that home visitation services unfold through a natural developmental process over time, consisting of sequential and overlapping stages that
determine what tasks can be intitiated at any given time and under what
circumstances. The understanding of the progression of these predictable stages—
with some variability depending on the particular case situation and the characteristics of staff—may help to provide information about the processes involved
in home visitation that are associated with this program's success at preventing
child abuse and neglect.

THE HEALTHY START PROGRAM OF HAWAII

The Healthy Start program of Hawaii is the model for the nationwide effort being
mounted by the National Committee to Prevent Child Abuse and Ronald
McDonald Children's Charities to create Healthy Families America. Nearly all

Hawaii's Healthy Start Program   57

50 states have now established task forces to advance the efforts of the Healthy Families initiative (Mitchel & Donnelly, 1993).

The Hawaii Healthy Start program had its origins in a 1975 demonstration by the Hawaii Family Stress Center—in collaboration with the Kapiolani Medical Center and the Hana Like Home Visitor Program—of the application of child abuse prevention ideas of Henry Kempe, M.D., former professor and chairman, Department of Pediatrics, University of Colorado Medical Center (Breakey & Pratt, 1993). In 1985, a 3-year demonstration project among high-risk parents in the Ewa district of the island of Oahu, implemented by Hawaii Family Stress Center with funding from the Hawaii Department of Health, Maternal and Child Health branch, led to an expansion of Healthy Start, involving direct service provision by seven private agencies throughout the state. The 14 Healthy Start sites are financed almost exclusively with state general funds which were about $7 million in 1993 (Breakey & Pratt, 1993). With this allocation, the program is available to serve approximately 52% of families with newborns across the state of Hawaii.

The sponsoring agencies within the Healthy Start statewide network, which include hospitals and community-based, comprehensive social service agencies, provide diverse organizational contexts for these home visitation programs. While all the Healthy Start programs focus on promoting access to health services and supporting parenting behaviors and relationship-based service strategies, the technical expertise and corporate culture of the sponsoring agency does shape the nature of modifications within the basic service mode. For example, a community-based agency, with a strong tradition of participation in grass-roots political activism, will view a parent advisory board as critical to program success and the promotion of a strengthened identity as a desired attribute of staff. Other affiliative settings may view the context of Healthy Start differently, though all must adhere to a basic set of criteria for services to families.

Though not a controlled demonstration, statistics related to the impact of Healthy Start have been impressive from the beginning. In the 1985 demonstration, 241 families were served with no cases of abuse and only four cases of neglect were found among families who were assessed at-risk using the validated Family Stress Checklist (Oskow, 1985). In addition, there was evidence of reduced family stress and of improved functioning within the target population served (Breakey & Pratt, 1991). Current data for the 2,254 families seen from July 1987 to July 1991 by Healthy Start and similar programs indicate that in 99.3% of target children, abuse was not confirmed. Abuse was confirmed for only 16 families. In addition, there was a 98.6% non-neglect rate among families receiving home visits (Hawaii State Department of Health, 1994).

Other outcome measures point to further positive effects of Healthy Start involvement. In a survey conducted from 1987 to 1990, 90% of 2-year olds were fully immunized as compared with total Hawaii statistics and recent data

58   *Nursing Care in a Violent Society: Issues and Research*

from a Carnegie Corporation study, which indicated that about 60% of 2-year-olds throughout the U.S. had not been immunized (Elmer-Dewitt, 1994). Ninety-five percent of the children had an identified primary health care provider. All children were enrolled in early periodic screening, diagnosis, and treatment (EPSDT) services, if eligible. Eighty-five percent of the children were developmentally age appropriate. Ninety percent of the mothers had received timely family planning information.

Other positive outcomes have been perceived by staff in the cooperating network of agencies. A large-scale evaluation is now under way that should further identify factors associated with both the processes and outcomes that have led to the favorable Healthy Start record.

STAFFING AND GENERAL PATTERN OF SERVICES

The selection of paraprofessional staff is made on the basis of those personal characteristics that are known to be related to the development of an effective helping relationship. In a national survey of home visitation programs, when staff were asked to identify essential home visitor attributes within their program, many identified communication and interpersonal skills, including maturity, warmth, and a nonjudgmental orientation (Wasik, 1993). Additional factors that guide Healthy Start staff selection include a capacity for empathy, concern for the feelings of children, ability to suppress personal views to allow a parent to explore life options, a belief that small children need to be nurtured, ability to cope with psychosocial stressors, a history of personally being nurtured as a child, and an enjoyment of people (Breakey, Uohara-Pratt, Morrel-Samuels, & Kolb-Latu, 1991). The foregoing are the qualities that are sought when screening applicants as Healthy Start home visitors. An extensive, formal training program builds upon these inherent capacities and is followed by a period of carefully supervised probationary service.

Training and supervision is essential with nonprofessionals who do not have the requisite skills to sort out the complex issues they confront when working with families who are difficult to engage and maintain in active service, as well as their own emotional reactivity to emotionally labile situations. A 5-week orientation training program, including didactic presentations as well as experiential training through visits to community agencies and through shadowing experienced home visitors, is offered to all paraprofessional staff. This training program includes the following broad content areas: an overview of secondary prevention and Healthy Start; basic skills and information necessary to effectively work with overburdened families; and the promotion of optimal infant development and parent-child interaction. An additional week of advanced training is provided 6 months following the initial program to reinforce and build on existing knowledge and skill, once staff have experienced the family support role. Further, the statewide training program provides funding

Hawaii's Healthy Start Program 59

for four half days of continuing education per year on an ongoing basis for each site (Breakey, Uohara-Pratt, Morrel-Samuels, & Kolb-Latu, 1991).

Some of the paraprofessionals are specially trained as early identification staff (EID) to examine medical records for indicators of risk and also to interview new mothers, using criteria from the previously cited Family Stress Checklist. This begins the process of identifying children at risk—and is thus appropriate for Healthy Start—at the time of birth. Among the criteria used to determine risk are such experiences as: childhood history of abuse or neglect for the mother or father; criminal, mental illness or substance abuse history; low self-esteem, isolation or poor coping and problem-solving abilities; multiple stressors from marital, occupational, housing and similar sources; anger management problems; and rigid or unrealistic expectations of the child by the mother; beliefs about discipline; and perceptions of the infant.

Those at risk are offered services for up to 5 years, if needed. Experience shows that services are accepted by about 90% of those who are found to be at risk (Breakey & Pratt, 1991). Because of high enrollment and the continuous and comprehensive nature of services, caseloads reach a maximum and eligible families cannot be offered services in certain locations and for varying periods of time. Also because of the intensity of the services, the plan is to keep caseloads to a maximum of 15 in new project sites, 20 cases in the second year and a maximum of 25 for third-year sites, when some families can be served less intensively and new families can be enrolled.

THE STAGES OF WORK WITH FAMILIES

The First Stage: Developing a Relationship and Offering Concrete Assistance

In the first stage of work with families, the support worker has four goals to accomplish:

1. facilitate a helping relationship;
2. define her or his (there are several male visitors) role with the family;
3. begin to teach families how to identify needs; and
4. begin to function as a broker to community services.

The first visit begins with attempts by the worker to create a positive relationship with the mother. To facilitate this connection, the worker describes the program and her role with the family. She usually expresses it in something like the following manner:

"I work with the Healthy Start program. I have new information about babies that I didn't know about when I was raising my kids. It can make being a mother easier, but not easy! Also you can look at me as your information center about this community. I live here, too, and I didn't know about WIC or the Well Baby Clinic before I started this job. I hope that you will learn to think of me as your "special" friend, someone here completely for you and the baby.

I am here to talk when you need to share something that concerns you. I know that it is hard to start with a new baby and to have so much on your mind."

While most families welcome this kind of expression of concern, others are less eager to respond to the offer of support. To the mothers who deny that they want information about the baby or someone to talk to, home visitors have learned to acknowledge their right to privacy, but also to attempt to sustain contact. They become comfortable in these circumstances saying: "It's OK that you feel like this right now, but would it be all right if I stop by next week to see how you're doing?" or "If your car breaks down and you need a ride to the doctor, just call."

Despite the best efforts of the workers to engage a family, about 10% to 15% of parents are unable to utilize support to cope with stressors. This is often difficult for the home visitors to accept. They sometimes assign self-responsibility to what they perceive as a failure to provide services. At this point, the supervisor can be helpful in interpreting the experience as that of a family exercising self-determination.

Most of the home visitors are residents of the communities they serve and some of them know what it is like to live with economic hardship. They are often emotionally unprepared, however, to confront the pervasively stressful life circumstances of the families served. The family who brings an infant home to a World War II Quonset hut without electricity or running water or to the back of a Toyota sedan or to a tent on a beach is coping with basic survival needs. In these situations, the home visitor often feels an urgent need to respond to the day-to-day chaotic events resulting from unstable housing, inadequate nutrition, and limited access to medical care. These events create the endless crises that drain the family's internal resources.

An important part of the initial alliance building with families is the family support worker's capacity to be substantially helpful from the beginning. This means providing immediate relief for some distressing problem. Such support could include helping a family secure AFDC (welfare) entitlements or a Department of Housing Section 8 (rent subsidy) waiver application, delivering a case of formula, or finding emergency food supplies for the family. It is understood that if true support is to be experienced by families, the immediate conditions that worsen poverty must be addressed.

Throughout this stage, the home visitor works to develop and sustain a helping relationship with the mother while she is attending to the family's concrete needs. Experience has shown that three factors are associated with facilitating a positive working alliance with families:

First, *empathic listening is a critical component of successful intervention with families.* Rogers (in Evans, 1975, p. 29) referred to this process as "to really stand in the client's shoes and to see the world from his (sic) vantage point" and to imply through actions that "I do really see how you feel." This is the most releasing kind of experience. Just being a good listener to a mother who feels confused by conflicting thoughts can at least temporarily relieve

Hawaii's Healthy Start Program   61

distress. Beyond the immediacy of the home visit the mother may begin to feel
free to say what she thinks, describe how she feels, and say what she wants,
which are all indicators of feelings of empowerment. Many Healthy Start
mothers have never had the experience described by Anderson (1979) of letting
out their thoughts and feelings without being judged as being right or wrong or
without being pressed for logic or clarity. Home visitors understand from their
training that effective listening is the way they express the depth of their
concern and let the mother know she is valued by another person.

Second, *the home visitation services seek to effect changes through an
enduring personal relationship* (Halpern, 1990). The home visitor uses a warm
and friendly style and an understanding of local cultures to facilitate reaching
out to the mother. She focuses conversation on significant events, social
activities, concerns, and personal problems in a way that is respectful and
accepting of a parent's individual life circumstances. As information is sought
about the family's situation, the key factor to facilitate a positive alliance is for
the home visitor to place an emphasis on enjoyment and nurturance of mother
and child while delaying active problem solving. Most essential, the home
visitor uses an understanding of the issues confronted by the family to forge a
positive connection with them.

Many of the home visitors identify strongly with the families they serve.
With a growing awareness of certain similarities in life experiences, they
become more open to using sensitive and timely self-disclosure in an effort to
strengthen their positions as positive role models.

A home visitor, working with a parenting teen who was terrified to tell her
mother she was pregnant again, told her client: "I know what it's like to be 19
years old with two infants." Another home visitor, whose mother died when she
was 7 years old, was able to share how she coped with a deep sense of longing
and loss with a client who was angry at having a remote, unavailable mother.
Another home visitor had a distressed mother who resisted joining a support
group, saying: "Why should I go and pour my heart out to strangers who don't
care?" The visitor was able to tell this mother that her daughter had lost a baby
and the worker found it helpful to be part of a support group. The client replied:
"I didn't think people like you who work with families needed help." Once the
value of such an experience was affirmed, the mother was able to follow
through with this successful referral. "When we use our life experiences to
show our clients that we are people like them, it makes us more real," said the
home visitor. "Then," she continued, "we are less threatening."

Third, *it is important to limit the role of paraprofessional staff.* To com-
pound the devastating problems of poverty, many parents haven't had the life
experiences that create or reinforce self-esteem or haven't a sense of being
loved, which can buffer chronic stress. They have lived a life of repeated
trauma, unmet needs, and limited social support.

As the home visitor begins to identify which problems the family is most
concerned about and what changes they would like to see in relation to these

62 *Nursing Care in a Violent Society: Issues and Research*

problems, she frequently becomes overwhelmed by the complexity of these situations. In light of this, the collaborative challenge for the supervisor and the home visitor is to specify the nature of the work with each family by identifying focal points of desired change and setting priorities among service goals.

This process of sorting out which client needs should be addressed in planned interventions is not an easy one. Halpern (1986) comments that the process of formulating a family's strengths and weaknesses in most home-based early intervention programs is gradual and incremental. The home visitor and the supervisor modify their initial information about family history as they observe how the parents interact with each other, the infant, and their social environment. Halpern (1986) states that among the keys to success of the diagnostic process are the quality of the observations of family functioning and the quality of the inferences drawn about intervention and support needs. This is best accomplished by maximizing activities related to psychosocial assessment and the development/revision of a service plan with families. All of these plans are based on observations of the home visitor, collaborative assessment by the supervisor, and use of instruments such as the Nursing Child Assessment Satellite Training Scales (NCAST), safe-home guidelines, and other such standardized tools (Breakey et al., 1991). Ideally, if funding were available, nurses would be utilized to provide neonatal assessments and information on infant care and preventive health practices as an adjunct service to this family support model.

Within the Healthy Start network, the supervisor is selected on the basis of demonstrated skills in the areas of professional counseling and supervision, a working knowledge of the principles of family support with economically disadvantaged populations and knowledge of maternal and child health, child development, and child abuse/interpersonal violence. While a qualified professional with these credentials could be drawn from the fields of social service, nursing, and public health, most of the professionals who seek and are selected for supervisory roles are social workers, marital and family therapists, and educational psychology counselors.

The Second Stage of Work with Families: Ongoing Assessment and Lowering Risk

During this stage, the home visitor applies knowledge of infant behavior to her working with mothers who demonstrate a wide range of maternal competencies. The home visitor learns to look at basic aspects of the parent–child relationship, within guidelines of the underlying theories of Ainsworth, Thomas and Chess, and Winnicott and others, and with some of the concrete assessment tools provided through the Healthy Start program. The visitor focuses on observable behaviors such as whether and under what circumstances a mother smiles at, vocalizes to, holds, and touches her infant. The visitor becomes more aware of how certain infant behaviors such as crying, sleeping, feeding, and soothability relate to parental handling. She begins to look at whether reciprocity or a positive rhythm exists between the parent and

Hawaii's Healthy Start Program 63

infant: Does the mother recognize cues and respond to the infant's needs, and does the baby in turn respond to the mother's actions? Is the tone of the parent–child interaction warm and loving or is there a shallow, mechanical attachment that is devoid of affect?

Many of the mothers enrolled in the program are eager to hear and talk about their infant's behavioral repertoire. They enjoy receiving age-related materials about infant development from the Healthy Start parent–infant interaction curriculum and apply it to their life with the baby. They quickly learn to utilize information on feeding, developmental milestones, and infant play. The home visitor knows that to acknowledge a mother's importance as her baby's "first and most important teacher" is to affirm her. "It lights up her face—she has more energy—if she feels important to her baby," recalled a home visitor of a mother who was growing in confidence and in ability to facilitate her child's growth.

For other mothers, however, the chronic stress within every aspect of family life drains their physical and emotional energy. This directs their attention away from consistent and nurturant infant caregiving and may even precipitate anger and violence-prone behaviors. In these situations, it is not uncommon for the home visitor to primarily focus interventions on the mitigation of stressful life circumstances. In this manner, the Healthy Start model of reducing parental stressors is implemented so that the mother has more energy to nurture her child.

The implementation dilemma during this stage, however, is the possibility of delay in addressing the developmental needs of the child until urgent family problems are resolved. When this happens, precious time may be lost for fostering attachment and observing or intervening in the parent–infant difficulties that may compromise infant development.

Barnard (Barnard, Woodruff, Provence, & Pawl, 1987), a consultant to the Healthy Start Program, speaks of two mottos that have guided her work with high-risk infants and the high-risk family. First, *infants can't wait*. Infancy is a critical period of human development. The child's behavior and caregiving interaction established in infancy has a long-term impact. Second, *all parents want to be good parents*. Despite a lack of knowledge or even in the face of their own personal problems, parents want to adequately care for their children. This is a positive assumption of parental good intent which undergirds the whole philosophy of Healthy Start.

As work progresses toward promoting attachment and optimal parent–child interaction, the growth of *both* the parent and the infant often needs to be facilitated. Support workers can help parents deal with personal limitations and social difficulties that may interfere with providing a protective, nurturing, and responsive home environment. On a routine basis, home visitors structure time with the family to allow for "teachable moments," when incidental learning about child development can occur. Parents are frequently delighted to hear about and observe their infant's unique capacities, including temperament qualities, ability to self-console, and social responsiveness. As parents are helped to read the individual differences of their infant, their ability to find pleasure in their infants and interact with them in loving ways is enhanced. Greenspan (1981) describes this reciprocal process of optimal caregiving as one of falling in love with the infant at the same time as it woos him/her to fall in love with the parent.

While nurses generally assist multi-risk families as primary agents of change, as in the case of a care coordinator in perinatal health settings or public health nursing roles, when they interface with the Healthy Start program they usually support the work of others through adjunct consultative roles during joint home visits or collaborative contacts with staff. Whatever nurses do, when they emphasize the best standards of maternal and child health practice, their contributions toward improving parent–child interaction, enhancing health care utilization, and promoting optimal child development are enormously helpful.

The Third Stage of Work: Consolidating Gains and Determining Ongoing High-Risk Parents

In this stage, home visitors become acutely aware that there is variability in the way individual families respond to supportive services. They recognize that family gains do not always accrue in a steady, upward course, that positive behavioral outcomes are often made in small steps, and that backsliding is common. In addition, they learn that when adults carry with them deep mental scars and a shattered human spirit from childhood without an opportunity to work through past hurts, such adults become locked into self-defeating patterns of behavior. For these families, movement through the Healthy-Start-level system in the expected 18–24 months to follow-up status on only a quarterly basis generally does not occur. Instead, they remain on the most intensive schedule of weekly home visits year after year.

Despite the extremely difficult life circumstances experienced by these families, the home visitor persists in her efforts to assist them. "We are here to back our clients no matter what they do," said one home visitor. "We are there to make sure that mom is safe and happy so that baby can be safe and happy," said another visitor with great conviction. The home visitor agrees to become the family's life line, someone to turn to, even if it is only for concrete needs. Home visitors have a sincere desire to make a difference, however small, and maintain some optimism about the family's future. They use the language of positive change in their work with all families, and most especially, with troubled, multi-problem families. They focus on the mother's strengths, her potential for more adaptive functioning, and whatever concrete steps she can take to realize her goals.

The supervisory guidelines that help to focus involvement with families during this stage are numerous. Healthy Start has found the following especially valuable: First, ambiguity in the home visitors' functions is reduced. The staff frequently feel the urgency of pressing life problems faced by families and

Hawaii's Healthy Start Program

want to meet basic needs. "At first our clients seem so needy. We are the only stable person in their lives; they cling to us," said one home visitor who was reflecting on her job. Over time, however, the home visitor learns to define the primary role as one of mobilizing clients to act on their own behalf. Visitors attempt to determine what clients are motivated to do and to differentiate between a mother who needs help for herself and a mother who needs parenting instruction. They help a client clarify problems, what her support system can do to help, and what responsibility she is able or willing to assume. The home visitors also need support as they identify obstacles that make client referrals unsuccessful.

Lerner and Halpern (1987) maintain that home visiting programs need to clearly specify the expectations laid on the visitors' shoulders in order to ensure that visitors will not overstep the limits of their expertise. These authors assert that programs need to focus on what home visitors do best—offer information, psychological support, and practical assistance.

Second, mutually defined goals that are manageable, achievable, and reasonable are set with the family. In prevention programs such as Healthy Start, the clients are not required to identify themselves as needing help nor are they required to enter into an agreement to work toward behavioral change (Bertacchi & Coplon, 1989). The only basic service requirement that is held out by Healthy Start is the expectation that clients allow the home visitor to enter their home and to make an attempt at interaction.

Third, once rapport is established, it is important to create opportunities and provide encouragement for families to take the often small—but threatening—steps forward. This is most critical in the area of parent–infant attachment. It is not enough that immunizations are updated; a primary health care provider is identified, and basic care to an infant is rendered, if they are done without parental warmth and concern. Without these qualities, the best interests of the child are not fully served.

Fourth, home visitors are assisted to maintain an amount of psychological distance and objectivity in their work with families. As the home visitors listen to the thoughts and feelings about emotionally laden life situations of the parents, they need to maintain a stance of neutrality. A home visitor who avoids reactivity to the family's anxiety, anger, and sadness will not become enmeshed during the process of helping.

Fifth, supervisors make it clear with the home visitor staff that limited client progress is not a reflection on the staff's competence. There is a tendency for the novice home visitor to personalize the onset of a client crisis. One home visitor reported that she used to worry that she did something wrong or didn't say the right thing and that her actions had precipitated the deterioration in a client's functioning. Changes take time. People are not failures or inadequate. Support workers are reminded that their families are doing the best they can considering what they have to work with.

The role of the home visitor when confronting families that test the limits and the boundaries defined by the program's structure, is to maintain the "holding

66   *Nursing Care in a Violent Society: Issues and Research*

environment" (Winnicott, 1965). The home visitor's consistent understanding of the parent's unmet needs acts as a buffer against the adverse qualities some parents may ascribe to the external world. As the parents' inner turmoil is expressed to the home visitor through disruptive actions that attempt to destroy the very interpersonal closeness they crave, the home visitor continues to be emotionally present with empathy rather than judgment.

Sixth, when staff attempt to be helpful with families confronting difficult life circumstances, these situations highlight the need to view the risks to healthy child development as multifaceted and demanding simultaneous attention to all forces in the caregiving environment. It is keenly recognized that the needs of families cannot be divided into discrete categories defined by traditional disciplinary boundaries. For example, in the case of a 16-year-old mother with a history of cocaine addiction prior to and during pregnancy, who is estranged from her family of origin and lives with the violence-prone father of her physically fragile infant, would the needs of this family be best met within the domain of medicine, nursing, social work, criminal justice, developmental psychology or a family support program? Given the complex nature of the needs and concerns of this family, it is of critical importance that the home visitor and the supervisor strive to develop a flexible and family-centered service plan that is based on collaboration among and between skilled service providers, with input from a range of disciplinary perspectives.

In the Healthy Start Child and Family Service Oahu teams, a master's level clinician is available to provide psychosocial assessment, crisis management, brief counseling, and case consultation services to both clients and home visitors on a selective basis. This clinician is a professional with training and experience in the human services, specifically in the areas of social work, counseling psychology, and marital and family therapy. Home visitors comment that it is a relief for them to access professional intervention with families who are having difficulty initiating or sustaining gains relative to service goals. Most of these situations involve difficulties with infant attachment, substance abuse, chronic psychiatric disturbance, and recurrent episodes of domestic violence that have been impervious or unresponsive to intervention.

Seventh, group services have been developed to interface with home visitation. Groups provide opportunities to create an extended community for young mothers. They can be focused in several ways:

(1) *Recreational Groups.* Celebrating a holiday or planning an outing to community sites (park, beach, zoo) that involve parents and children interacting together in a playful, casual way, is a positive experience for families.

(2) *Structured Support Groups.* Staff invest their energy in the process of creating activities and encouraging participation by parents who might otherwise choose to remain alone. Whether the group is painting T-shirts, perfecting their hula or preparing sushi, there is spontaneous interaction that develops among the parents. The staff model social skills, respond to individuals in a nurturing way, and facilitate group interaction.

Hawaii's Healthy Start Program   67

(3) *Psychoeducational Groups*. A focus on topics of concern to mothers, such as their role as parents, intimate relationships, and their sense of self, directs the interaction within these groups. The groups, facilitated by professional staff with home visitor participation, provide a source of nurturance and self-esteem that enables a mother to begin to explore her own behavior. Self-examination and taking responsibility for what they feel, think, and do can be threatening without the support and growth derived from the group. In groups, however, parents can be more open to learning communication skills, receiving positive reinforcement for behavior change, and solving everyday problems.

(4) *Simultaneous Play Groups*. These are organized for a multi-age group of children, 6 months to 5 years, leaving their mothers free to have an adult experience independent of them. At first, some mothers are reluctant to let go of clinging infants or are fearful that their toddlers will become disruptive with other children in the play groups. Over time, however, mothers learn to relax and engage in other activities provided at Healthy Start sites.

SUMMARY

In the 1990s, service systems must draw upon the interventive frameworks that are sensitive to family concerns, build on family strengths, enhance family functioning, and create new competencies within families. This can best be accomplished through an interdisciplinary service approach that fosters communication and collaboration among and between skilled professionals in the best interest of developing a family-focused plan to guide problem identification and strategies for intervention.

The Healthy Start program has proven effective in preventing abuse in nearly all families served. The key component of service is the provision of home visiting by family support workers. Experience has taught that the stages in the work with families described here can be understood by both service providers and their supervisors in such a manner as to help provide guidelines in the work with high-risk families. The work can be intense but highly rewarding as children are seen to truly get a Healthy Start in life.

REFERENCES

Ainsworth, M. (1973). The development of infant-mother attachment. In B. Caldwell, & H. Ricciuti (Eds.), *Review of child development research*. (Vol. 3, p. 159). Chicago: University of Chicago Press.

Anderson, G. D. (1979). Enhancing listening skills for work with abusing parents. *Social Casework, 60,* 602-608.

Barnard, K., Woodruff, G., Provence, S., Pawl, J. (1987). Working with infants, toddlers, and their families: What we do and how we keep going. *Zero-to-Three, National Center for Clinical Infant Programs, 7,* 13-17.

68   *Nursing Care in a Violent Society: Issues and Research*

Bertacchi, J., & Coplon, J. (1989). The professional use of self in prevention: *Zero-to-Three. National Center for Clinical Infant Programs. 9*(4), 1-7.

Breakey, G., Uohara-Pratt, B., Morrel-Samuels, S., & Kolb-Latu, D. (1991). *The Healthy Start Manual.* Hawaii State Department of Health, Maternal and Child Health Branch.

Breakey, G., & Pratt, B. (1991). Healthy Growth for Hawaii's "Healthy Start": Towards a systematic statewide approach to the prevention of child abuse and neglect. *Zero-to-Three. 11*(4), 16-22.

Breakey, G., & Pratt, B. (1993). Healthy Start home visiting: Hawaii's approach. *The American Professional Society on the Abuse of Children Advisor, 6*(4), 7-8.

Daro, D. (1988). *Confronting child abuse.* New York: Free Press.

Daro, D. (1993). Special Issue: Home visitation and preventing child abuse. *The American Professional Society on the Abuse of Children Advisor, 6*(4), 1, 4.

Elmer-Dewitt, P. (April 18, 1994). The crucial years. *Time,* p. 68.

Evans, R. J. (1975). *Carl Rogers: The man and his ideas.* New York: E.P. Dutton.

Greenspan, S. L. (1981). *Psychopathology and adaptation in infancy and early childhood, principles of clinical diagnosis and preventive intervention.* New York: International Universities Press, Inc.

Halpern, R. (1986). Home-based early intervention; dimensions of current practice. *Child Welfare, 65*(4), 387-398.

Halpern, R. (1990). Community-based early intervention. In S. J. Meisels & J. P. Shonkoff (Eds.), *Handbook of early childhood intervention* (pp. 469-498). Cambridge, England: Cambridge University Press.

Hawaii State Department of Health, Family Health Services Division, Maternal and Child Health Branch. (1994). Outcomes for the Hawaii Healthy Start Program; revised: Author.

Larner, M., & Halpern, R. (1987). Lay home visiting programs: Strengths, tensions and challenges. *Zero-to-Three. National Center for Clinical Infant Programs. 8*(1), 1-7.

Mitchel, L., & Donnelly, A. C. (1993). Healthy Families America: Building a national system. *American Professional Society on the Abuse of Children Advisor, 6*(4), 9-10: 27.

Musick, J. S., & Stott, F. M. (1990). Paraprofessionals, parenting and child development: Understanding the problem and seeking solutions. In B. J. Meisels & J. P. Shonkoff (Eds.), *Handbook of early childhood intervention* (pp. 651–667). Cambridge, England: Cambridge University Press.

Olds, D. L., Henderson, C. R., Jr., Tatelbaum, R., & Chamberlain, R. (1986). Improving the life-course development of socially disadvantaged mothers: A randomized trial of nurse home visitation. *American Journal of Public Health, 78,* 1436-1445.

Oskow, B. (1985). Implementation of a Family Stress Checklist. *Child Abuse and Neglect, 9,* 405-410.

Seitz, V., Rosenbaum, L., & Apfel, N. (1985). Effects of family support intervention: A ten-year follow-up. *Child Development, 56,* 376-391.

Thomas, A., & Chess, S. (1984). Genesis and evolution of behavioral disorders: From infancy to early adult life. *American Journal of Psychiatry, 141,* 1-9.

U.S. Department of Health and Human Resources, Office of Human Development Services, U.S. Advisory Board on Child Abuse and Neglect. (1990). *Child abuse and neglect: Critical first steps in response to a national emergency.* Washington, DC: Author.

Wasik, B. (1993). Staff issues for home visiting programs. *The Future of Children, Home Visiting, 3,* Winter, 140-157.

Hawaii's Healthy Start Program   69

Werner, A., & Smith, R. S. (1982). *Vulnerable but invincible: A longitudinal study of resilient children and youth.* New York: McGraw-Hill.
Willis, D., Holden, E., & Rosenberg, M. (1992). *Prevention of child maltreatment: Developmental and ecological perspectives.* New York: John Wiley & Sons.
Winnicott, D. W. (1965). *The maturational process and the facilitating environment.* New York: International Universities Press.

Acknowledgments: The authors wish to thank Kay Foy, Loretta Fuddy, Betsy Uohara-Pratt, and the Healthy Start home visitors and supervisors for insights and suggestions which were helpful to the creation and revision of this chapter. This publication was adapted from a paper presented by Vicki Wallach at the First Healthy Families American Annual Conference, February 5–7, 1992, Honolulu, Hawaii.

5

The Psychological Impact of Caring for Victims of Violence: Vicarious Traumatization

Carol R. Hartman

Vicarious traumatization is a phenomenon that recognizes that the exposure of persons, other than the victim, to the specifics of trauma material or the reenactment of traumatic experiences transmits the emotionally laden aspects of the original violence and thus is a source of emotional arousal and distress for the nurse working with victims of violence. This source of emotional arousal shapes the underlying approach—avoidance dynamic of countertransference responses that strain the empathic connection necessary for a safe and constructive nurse–patient relationship. Case consultation and supervision are necessary to protect the integrity of the nurse–patient relationship. The current isolating changes in the work setting cut the nurse off from needed support and guidance in working with victims of violence. The emotional risks inherent in working with victims of violence require that the nurse seek professional support for the interpersonal aspects of practice.

A former patient enters a clinic and shoots to kill his therapist, a social worker, and another staff member. A 32-year-old woman, admitted because of a seizure disorder and back injury, screams at the nurses attending her. She berates them, calls them incompetent, and is reduced to tears. A nurse in the emergency room receives the battered body of an 8-month-old child; he dies. His young parents are arraigned for sexual abuse and for beating the baby. The nurse finds it increasingly difficult to go to work on this unit and requests a transfer to another unit. A therapist who has worked long and hard with a patient informs the patient of her impending marriage. The patient becomes enraged and levels a lawsuit against the therapist, claiming sexual abuse and abandonment. After years of legal involvement, the therapist realizes she can no longer take patients with a history of sexual abuse.

Locations and length of the professional relationship vary in these examples; what does not vary is that in each situation the patient has a complex history of experiencing abuse and violent actions. Other commonalities are that professional nurses in these situations are privy to violent past experiences either through the behavior of the patient toward the nurse or because of the consequences of the violent behavior toward others.

72   *Nursing Care in a Violent Society: Issues and Research*

The consequences of patients telling their trauma stories or their reenactment of these experiences with others are at the basis of what is known as secondary traumatization (Danieli, 1985; Figley,1988; Pynoos & Nader, 1988; Solomon, 1990) or vicarious traumatization. Vicarious traumatization was introduced into the clinical literature by McCann and Pearlman (1990) and avoids some of the confusion of meaning associated with the notion of retraumatization in the process of helping. For example, a rape victim is often 'secondarily' traumatized by the legal system when the victim is made out to be responsible for the rapist's behavior. What is specific to the concept of vicarious traumatization is the recognition that the exposure of persons, other than the victim, to the specifics of trauma material or the reenactment of traumatic experiences transmits the emotionally laden aspects of the original violence and thus is a source of emotional arousal and distress for those persons. In turn, this emotional arousal can have parallel effects on the biological processes of the receiver as the prolonged arousal has on the victim. Therefore, victims of violence who come to the nurse for various forms of help are also a source of potential distress for the nurse. Nurses' reactions to this trauma information on both biological and psychological levels result in nontherapeutic responses and patterns of interaction within the nurse–patient relationship. Nontherapeutic patterns are marked by behaviors that overinvolve the nurse or result in the nurse's withdrawal from the patient. These behaviors adversely affect the empathic connection necessary for the therapeutic outcome of the nurse–patient relationship.

EVIDENCE FOR VICARIOUS TRAUMATIZATION

Literature in the field of traumatology has increasingly demonstrated that the effects of traumatic life events go beyond those who directly experience them. Utterback and Caldwell (1989), in investigating the aftermath of campus violence, noted that families, friends, and bystanders who did not experience the trauma itself, had debilitating symptoms similar to those of the victims. The carryover of trauma information from one generation to another has been noted by numerous researchers involved in the study of Holocaust survivors and their families (Danieli, 1985) and veterans and their families (Figley, 1988). Solomon (1990) found that wives of Israeli veterans with posttraumatic stress disorder (PTSD) experienced increased psychiatric symptomatology, somatic complaints, and loneliness. Others have noted that symptoms in traumatized children appear to activate fear and terror in other children (Eth & Pynoos, 1985). Kelley (1992) and Hartman, Burgess, Burgess and Kelley (1991) report on the symptoms presented by parents of children who were sexually abused in nursery schools and who went to court. Kelley reported that both mothers and fathers manifested symptoms of PTSD over a lengthy period of time and

Vicarious Traumatization

that the intensity of these symptoms was greater for those parents whose children were exposed to the most damaging sexual abuse. In a secondary analysis of the interaction of symptoms within the triad of the mother, father, and child, data suggest that the child's symptoms impact on the mother and the symptoms of the parents interact with each other,that is, mother influences father and vice versa (Hartman, Burgess, Burgess, & Kelley, 1992).

With regard to those working with trauma survivors, a variety of reports underscore the debilitative effects of this work. Sleep disturbance and nightmares have been reported by a variety of investigators exploring the impact of trauma work on providers (Danieli, 1984; Langer, 1987). Mollica (1988), working with his staff who deal with Southeast Asian populations, stated that "therapists become infected with their clients' hopelessness" (p. 300). McCann and Pearlman (1990) studied therapists, and noted that the symptom presentation and behaviors of the therapists were distinct from the symptoms of burnout. In Munroe's study (1991) of therapist's working with combat veterans, intrusive thoughts of the veterans' trauma stories and withdrawal from the veterans was significantly related to the amount of combat exposure in their clients. One of the best predictors of symptom development in traumatized individuals is the intensity and duration of exposure (Gleser, Green, & Winget, 1981; Hartsough, 1988). In the extensive work done by Kluft (1989) and Putnam (1989) with arranging therapeutic settings for dealing with complex cases of sexual and physical abuse resulting in dissociative disorders, special care was taken to provide focused supervision and consultation to the nursing staff. These units are designed to assist the nurse and staff to deal with their reactions to patients and to prevent the debilitating effects of vicarious traumatization (Kluft, 1994).

The foregoing documentation of vicarious traumatization in therapists and, in particular, nursing staff on units dealing with populations of trauma patients, suggests that we cannot ignore that working with victims of violence poses a potential occupational hazard. Nursing has not ignored the psychological impact of caring for those in pain and dying. There has been a tradition of research focusing on stress in the working environment and its relationship to nursing care (Hinshaw & Astwood, 1984; Jacobson & McGrath, 1983; Norbeck, 1986; Stanton & Schwartz, 1954; Vachon, 1987). In Vachon's (1987) seminal study of stress in the care of the critically ill, the dying, and the bereaved, she notes in her chapter on the psychological manifestions of stress that younger physicians and nurses (12% of 600 caregivers in a hospital setting) reported errors in clinical judgment as a result of the stress they were experiencing. Fewer errors were reported by the older nurses and physicians and none by other providers. While this may be consistent with the literature (Livingston &Livingston, 1984), Vachon suggests that older nurses and physicians may be reluctant to report errors. She further recounts the comments of nurses and physicians struggling with the impact of mistakes on their psychological well-

74 *Nursing Care in a Violent Society: Issues and Research*

being. In addition to issues in judgment, she stated that 63% of the nurses reported symptoms of depression, grief, guilt, helplessness, inadequacy, anger, and irritability.

The current findings in populations of care providers dealing with known trauma populations and past information about nurses in stressful working situations make it imperative that when we consider nursing practice with such victims, we have a basis for understanding vicarious traumatization. The first step in this understanding is to attend to the acute as well as cumulative effects of the heightened emotional arousal associated with trauma information and its impact on the biological, behavioral, and psychological systems of the nurse.

THE BIOLOGICAL, BEHAVIORAL, AND PSYCHOLOGICAL RESPONSES TO VIOLENCE

The symptom complex of psychological responses to violence is understood within five broad categories of responses that support the hypothesis of altered central nervous system dysregulation (Giller, 1990; van der Kolk & Saporta, 1993). These are: (1) *Intrusive Symptoms*: flashbacks, vivid nightmares of traumatic events, preoccupation with traumatic events, thinking of events in the face of reminders in the environment of the events; (2) *Avoidance Symptoms*: purposeful avoidance of reminders of the events, avoiding thinking of the events; (3) *Hyperautonomic Arousal Symptoms*: heightened startle reflex, constant vigilance, startling to neutral stimuli, sleep disruption, alterations in pain response, increased heart rate; (4) *Numbing Symptoms*: detachment from emotions, memory lapses, lapses in sense of time, detachment from surroundings from either internal or external reminders of the events; and (5) *Distortions of the Self-System*: alterations in ability to soothe self, self-consistency, self-cohesion, self-monitoring, sustaining self-esteem, and sensing oneself as part of a social community (Buie, 1994; Friedman, 1993; Herman, 1992; Horowitz, 1976). These symptoms are best understood as basic disruptions of biological systems and neural networking and the emerging behavioral and psychological systems (van der Kolk & Sapata, 1993; Hartman & Burgess, 1993).

Biological research indicates that in the face of violent events for either victim or witness, such as sexual and physical abuse, murder or assault with a gun, the alarm system is overridden and changed in its capacity to return to flexible functioning. Changes appear in the alteration of functions in the brain stem that relate to and connect with the limbic system and neural networking systems involved in higher-order behavioral and psychological functions. The changes linked to limbic functioning are central to memory, learning and emotional control, sleep, hormonal and immune regulation, and attachment subsystems. These systems are basic to patterns of interpersonal functioning, intrapersonal functioning, and sense of integrity. Many of the neurotransmit-

Vicarious Traumatization

ters essential to learning, memory, and the integration of experience are altered under the biological forces of overriding trauma, resulting in neurostructural changes that are not amenable to change through normal exposure to constructive events. There have been permanent alterations in these complex, interrelated systems. These changes result in altered biological responsiveness and behavioral and psychological responses. Memory and mechanisms for learning, particularly interpersonal and emotional learning, are altered in such a manner as to increase a sense of fragmentation and separation from oneself and the community of others. These alterations are manifested by dissociation within and between these systems. Dissociation is experienced physiologically, behaviorally, and psychologically, and, ultimately, socially and spiritually (Hartman & Burgess, 1988; 1993).

In numerous clinical reports and in-depth interviews with professionals who have worked with trauma patients, we begin to document symptoms and behaviors that parallel those of trauma victims and are the hallmarks of countertransference in the provider (Hartman & Jackson, 1994; McCann & Pearlman, 1990; Munroe et al., 1994; Wilson & Lindy, 1994).

Professionals working in environments such as emergency rooms, disaster relief, and prisons, and those working with victims and perpetrators of violence, report an array of symptoms and behaviors and ideational changes in themselves. There is *increased physiological and physical reaction*. The symptoms associated with autonomic arousal are rapid heart rate at resting, somatic reactions, sleep disturbances (particularly REM abnormalities), agitation, inattention, drowsiness, and uncontrolled and unintended emotional displays. These reactions occur with patients and are carried over into the private life of the caregiver. *Emotional reactions* include irritability, annoyance or disdain; anxiety and fear reactions; depression and sadness; anger, rage, and hostility; detachment, denial, and avoidance; sadistic/masochistic reactions; voyeuristic and sexualized reactions; and confusion, psychic overload, overwhelmed reactions, and guilt. These reactions often are responded to with shame and embarrassment as they are manifested in interactions with patients, coworkers, and families. The reactions underscore the emotional dysregulation. *Psychological reactions* are detachment, overuse of intellectualization, rationalization, isolation, denial, minimization, and fantasy. Another complex response is overidentification with the patient with increased use of psychological defenses such as projection, introjection, and denial.

A last grouping of signs of vicarious traumatization and resultant countertransference includes behavioral symptoms that may or may not be in the conscious awareness of the provider, for example, forgetting appointments, lapse of attention, parapraxes (distorted perceptions of the patient), loss of empathy, hostility, and anger toward patient, relief when the patient misses an appointment or a wish that the patient not show up for appointments, denial of feelings, denial of need for supervision or consultation regarding the patient, a self-centered belief that one has a special "gift" for working with a certain

76 *Nursing Care in a Violent Society: Issues and Research*

population of victims of violence, overconcern and/or identification with the patient, psychic numbing or emotional constriction, self-medication of numbing (increased use of drugs and alcohol); loss of professional boundaries during work with patient and reactions where the professional takes on the total experience of the patient, or where the professional takes on a more or less positive vantage point of the patient's plight (such as that of the protector or rescuer); or the professional takes on a complementary vantage point of the patient, where the professional can be the punisher, the abusive parent. These increased patterns of involvement are also associated with intense preoccupation with the patient (can't stop thinking about the patient), dreams and disturbed sleep, being easily reminded of the patient when not intending to think about him or her.

The factors indicative of symptoms of vicarious traumatization are also the signals of what is called countertransference. The terms *transference* and *countertransference* traditionally refer to the impact that the therapist and patient have on one another. When specific trauma information affects the therapist, we see the array of symptoms outlined above that parallel the trauma response in the victim. The symptoms alert us to the fact that the provider is under stress and they point to the fact that breaches in the professional relationship are a function of the trauma-specific information and behavior. In addition, the behaviors of the care provider fall within the broad categories outlined for post-traumatic stress disorder: intrusive thoughts, avoidance behaviors, autonomic arousal, numbing, and disturbances in self-system and interpersonal relationships (Danieli, 1981; Haley, 1974; Hartman & Jackson 1994; Wilson & Lindy, 1994).

It is important that nurses are able to protect and provide safety for themselves without compromising the therapeutic relationship. While these symptoms and behaviors alert us to the potential for real lapses in an empathic and therapeutic response to the trauma patient, they are, first and foremost, indicators that nurses need to take time out for themselves and reflect on what is impacting on them. One first and important step is to understand the phenomenon of transference and countertransference reactions as inevitable, expected, and natural in the face of relating to people who are attempting to assimilate overwhelming life events. When nurses reach out to support such people, nurses are also exposed to emotional risk. An understanding of the natural aspects of responses to violence in both victims and nurses is essential to the next step of analyzing the processes of the nurse–patient relationship.

TRANSFERENCE AND COUNTERTRANSFERENCE WHEN PSYCHOLOGICAL TRAUMA FROM PERSONAL VIOLENCE IS AT THE ROOT

The linking of vicarious traumatization to the processes of transference and countertransference brings the latter concepts within the realm of normal and

Vicarious Traumatization

expected adaptive reactions to overwhelming life events. The importance of the link is for the nurse to realize that the trauma information (be it the details of the trauma or its reenactment in the interpersonal process) can have a contagious effect regardless of the particular characteristics of the nurse. A review of the concepts of transference and countertransference puts this link into a contemporary perspective.

The concepts of transference and countertransference came into being with the advent of psychoanalysis (Freud, 1910–1912). Transference, the reenactment of patterns of relating to primary people in one's past within the relationship to the analyst, was the cornerstone of the ultimate event to be attended to in the analytic process. The response of the analyst in a likewise fashion (having strong negative or positive reactions toward the patient), whether overt or covert, was seen initially as a "nuisance" to the analyst. Basically, when aware of such a reaction, the analyst was to keep it to him/herself. The noncommittal stance, with exception of the "interpretations" of the analyst, was critical to the work and to the purity of the information coming from the patient. Analysts and students of therapy as early as 1924, however, believed the therapeutic relationship was anything but a one-sided projection emanating from the patient (Sullivan, 1953). For many of these more contemporary students of behavior and therapy, the process of acting and reacting in the therapeutic situation was a natural process. A major question was whether the analyst or therapist should disclose his/her reactions to the patient, and, if so, to what end. The second major question was whether countertransference was useful to the therapy and, if it was, in what way; if it was not, the therapist was left to seek therapy for him/herself. For many whose theoretical orientation was that of an interactionist, countertransference held out much more as a way of learning about what the patient was trying to express and have understood. There was agreement, too, that if it was not addressed by the therapist, countertransference could lead to problems in the therapeutic relationship. Often these problems manifested themselves in exploitive relationships or premature abandonment of therapy by either the patient or the therapist (see reviews by Racker, 1968; Slatker, 1987).

The links between the phenomenon of vicarious traumatization and countertransference/transference draws clinical attention to the categories of behaviors that the nurse must address in working with trauma victims. From the research and literature coming from those doing therapy with trauma victims, it is now recognized that behaviors carried over to the therapist represent not only issues reminiscent of the direct victim experience itself but of a complex array of defensive strategies to ward off dangers in reengaging in a trusting relationship. The reactions of the provider, in turn, manifest strong personal reactions to the patient, whether those reactions are directly revealed or not. It is no longer an argument whether transference and countertransference exist in this broader definition of these concepts. Rather, the reality of the process presents a challenge to recognize and learn from these reactions and deal with

78   *Nursing Care in a Violent Society: Issues and Research*

them so that an empathic connection can be maintained (Wilson & Lindy, 1994).

A therapeutic empathic connection is manifested in the capacity to confirm others' experiences, desires, conflicts, etc., without losing objectivity or a sense of oneself, and through verbal and nonverbal behavior to communicate the 'understanding.' Empathy in and of itself is an amoral process but is critically shaped by the values and parameters of a therapeutic relationship. In the realm of human relationships, empathy generally provides for connection and a basis of emotional understanding that when reasonably maintained, provides the basic support for patients to: do the work of processing what happened to them, reduce the personal fragmentation that now renders them limited in their lives, and alter distortions arising in interpersonal relationships.

While the nurse–patient relationship is central to all of the roles in which nurses find themselves, the requirement to study the dynamics of this relationship within the varied contextual climates of the counseling is less familiar. Further, the nature of these various contexts for the nurse–patient relationship does not always lend itself to unearthing the patient's personal information that might assist nurses in comprehending what they themselves are experiencing. Nurses in a variety of settings often exhibit excellent self-control with regard to their reactions to challenging behaviors on the part of patients. Over time, however, this gets more difficult as the nurses are exposed either to repeated loss, pain, and suffering or to the terror and anxiety expressed in the repetitions and defensive styles of relating. Given the broader conceptualization and recognition of the transference and countertransference processes, all nurses must be ready to learn about this aspect of the nurse–patient relationship. A useful model in understanding this process is presented by Wilson and Lindy (1994). Highlights of this model are presented below.

Typology of Countertransference

Following from a more specific understanding of trauma information's central role in the phenomenon of transference and countertransference, Wilson and Lindy (1994) suggest two broad countertransference reaction styles of the therapist: Type I (CTR) avoidance and Type II (CTR) overidentification. In Type I CTR there is Empathic Withdrawal, marked by a blank screen façade, intellectualization, and misperception of dynamics, and Empathic Repression, marked by withdrawal, denial of the patient's claim, and distancing from the patient. In Type II CTR there is Empathic Disequilibrium, marked by uncertainty, vulnerability, and unmodulated affect, and Empathic Enmeshment, marked by loss of boundaries, overinvolvement, and reciprocal dependency.

Factors within both the patient and nurse play a role in shaping the countertransference, as do factors within the social context bearing on the nurse–patient relationship. These can be summarized as follows: (1)The nature

Vicarious Traumatization 79

of the trauma story (natural disaster vs. interpersonal violence); (2) personal factors in the nurse (e.g., own history of trauma, defensive style, knowlege about trauma, beliefs regarding the victim and trauma endured); (3) institution/organizational factors (e.g., administrative support for programs for trauma victims, resources both for the patient and the nurse); and (4) specific factors in the patient (e.g., type of event experienced, gender, level of traumatic injury, defensive style, and reenactment patterns).

For most nurses, their contacts with victims of violence will not be within the role of counseling to resolve the psychological impact of the trauma experiences. Rather, the nurse's role will be within the context of the immediate aftermath of the events themselves. Such situations are: emergency service in the face of physical assault and rape; discovery of abuse such as spousal abuse; or some phase of the victim's amnesia for the trauma experience where the victim becomes difficult to help. An example is a woman who becomes hysterical as the nurse attempts to do a pelvic examination. Both the nurse and patient are unaware of the origins of the patient's behavior, for example, being held down and raped by her pediatrician as a child. In these situations the nurse, physician, or other 'helpers' are perplexed by the behavior. The highly defensive and frantic behavior of the victim bombards the senses of the nurse. There is hyperarousal, increased sense of helplessness, and anger, and no convenient outlet for these defensive emotions. The trauma information communicated in a defensive style, without understanding, creates many avenues of strain with the nurse. The affective arousal, if not attenuated, contributes to empathic strain. In turn, the nurse adds self-pressure in trying not to act in an 'unprofessional' manner with the patient. The nurse is now confronted with a challenge to her/his own self-integrity as a professional.

Examples of CTR I and CTR II

Certainly, the strong affective arousal is understandable when a beaten and battered individual enters an emergency room. The impact of this arousal is less obvious when, for example, a male nurse recognizes the woman as having been in the emergency room before, referred to a shelter, and given assistance in getting a restraining order against her husband, only to return to him, and now again to the emergency room. The nurse presents himself with a noncommittal appearance, attends to the wounds, collaborates with the physician, and then discharges the woman, home. He does not inquire as to her safety or to her need for follow-up services. His avoidance corresponds to Type I CTR. In contrast is Type II CTR, where a female nurse is not sure what to do, feels helpless, ministers to a battered woman, and feels too emotional to talk with her but in desperation gives her her own home phone number so the patient might get information on shelters without the husband knowing.

In the first example, the male nurse reflected on his care to this woman and his concern regarding his work in the setting. He did not expect to deal with these female victims of violence and he does not like the work. He was defensive about his stand, commenting on how angry he is at these women who do nothing to help themselves. In the second example, the female nurse reported she could not sleep that night and wonders, with mixed feelings, whether the woman will call, and, if so, what she will do. In both situations, the nurses fear and avoid consulting their supervisors, feeling embarrassed and unsure of the response they might get. Rather both, now emotionally overloaded, isolate themselves and attempt to forget their experiences. These emergency room nurses reported disruption in sleep and feeling isolated and cut off from others; they were seriously considering changing their job setting.

A more complex example of the dynamics of transference and countertransference is the following interaction between admissions room nurses and personnel and ward nurses in a local psychiatric hospital. We learn how defensive role shifts create sensory overload for the nurse. A patient phoned before coming into the hospital, inquiring about admission. She explained that she was a survivor of sexual abuse and was being plagued with flashbacks. She related she was fearful of hospitals, having had bad experiences in them, but felt she needed the protection of the hospital now. She was given instructions as to where the evaluation unit was located.

Upon arrival, the patient became upset because access to the evaluation unit required that she enter through locked units. She became frightened and expressed her fears and doubts to the friends that accompanied her to the hospital. When a female clerk approached her for identifying information, the patient became defensive and complained about the locked doors. When the clerk further informed her that her evaluation would take place on a locked unit upstairs, the patient's anxiety increased. The clerk became visibly upset and perplexed; she retreated to her office. A few minutes later another woman arrived and introduced herself as the nurse on the admission unit.

As the patient lamented the 'prison-like' quality of the institution, her rage at locked units, and the distrust she felt of the total situation, the nurse patiently explained to her that the decision to continue with the evaluation process and entry into the hospital was up to the patient. When these verbal interventions resulted in the patient quieting and lowering her voice, the nurse relaxed. When the patient picked up a minute point and returned to a defensive posture, the nurse became tense. Eventually, the patient agreed to go the evaluation unit. To get to the unit, she had to walk past rooms that were obviously empty, quiet rooms for disturbed patients. This escalated the patient's defensive anxiety and she wavered as to whether to continue with the evaluation. The nurse was visibly relieved to turn the evaluation process over to another nurse and a physician. The patient sensed the defensiveness of the staff and began to confront them with their defensive behavior and their lack of sensitivity as to

Vicarious Traumatization

what it took for her to come on the unit and trust them. Both the nurse and physician found words that at one moment calmed the patient and at the next stirred in her the deepest distrust and defensiveness. The strain on the team was apparent and they began to take more time out for themselves, making time for the patient to have a small lunch and become familiar with the surroundings. Initially, the patient felt comforted by this but eventually she became suspicious and distrustful.

At least 2 hours transpired before the physician came in for the focused part of the evaluation. The patient informed the physician that she had little trust in psychiatrists and felt that through the years they had harmed her more than helped her. As she and the physician gained a level of rapport, time came for the physician to call, with the patient's permission, the neurologist who was managing her seizure condition. The physician returned and informed the patient that her neurologist was not on call, but he talked with the covering physician. The patient, in great anger, berated the physician for 'betraying her confidence' in speaking to a physician other than the one she agreed to. A great deal of time was needed to regain rapport and clarity as to whether the patient wished to continue with the evaluation and be admitted. Angrily and defensively she continued the process. Time elapsed before she was taken over to the ward. During this time, the evaluation team was stressed and angry with the patient. They were delayed in the admission procedure which increased the tension in the patient.

On the way to her assigned ward, the patient was taken through an underground tunnel. Two things happened simultaneously: She had a series of flashbacks of early abuse experiences and a seizure. When she arrived on the unit she was terrified and was incapacitated because she was dazed from the seizure. Her friend tried to explain to the nurses on the unit that she was having a seizure as well as flashbacks and that her slurred speech and dazed expression were physical signs of the type of seizure disorder. The two nurses insisted the patient had dissociated and they would take care of her. They then walked away and the patient grabbed her friend's hand explaining how terrified she was and that she could not be taken into tunnels. In a weakened state, she lamented her agreement to come into the hospital.

At this point another nurse came to the patient and identified herself as the patient's nurse for the afternoon. She took the patient to her room where, in the admission process, she learned of the patient's fears of the tunnel, the seizues and the flashbacks. The nurse spent over an hour with the patient and as she left, the patient's anxiety was less and she went to sleep. Upon awakening, she wanted to see her assigned nurse and when the nurse came, the patient began to again express her fear and anxiety. The nurse listened but then had to leave. The patient responded with anger, raising her voice. The nurse pointed out it was time for her to leave, that she had other patients to attend to but that she would be back. Though the patient tried to contain herself, her demanding attitude and accusatory behavior spilled over to other staff members. Soon the staff was impatient and angry with the patient and one staff member stated that if the patient did not calm down they would put her in four-point restraints. This terrified the patient.

The next day the physician in charge talked with her. She felt heard. He did not find her reactions 'paranoid' and without grounds in past reality. He reduced restriction and gave her freedom to leave the unit at will. She settled down and felt able to accept hospitalization but now felt her 'ally' was the physician and those to mistrust were the 'nurses' on the unit. By the end of 2 days, the physician suggested that the patient leave the hospital because the staff could not handle her.

This example captures all of the subtleties of working with the reenactment of past traumas and the now deep and permeating distrust of others. The manifest distrust pulls staff into alliances or alienated positions with the patient, or drives the staff into conflict with one another. The increased physiological arousal in staff is responded to by threatening behavior toward the patient.

The reader is asked in reading this abbreviated process of interactions to acknowledge the emotional shift toward the patient. One can identify being pushed away and pulled toward the patient. There is an increase in self-criticism and criticism of others. The physician's position may have stimulated a sense of betrayal within the nursing staff. The movement toward Type I CTR and Type II CTR becomes clear. The mounting tension in the nurses is responded to with defensive and threatening behavior in interactions with the patient. The staff becomes the abuser, or the person abandoning the patient or an ally in a split between personnel where one becomes the comforter and rescuer, only to betray the position when other demands take the person away from the patient. At that point, terror and rage are released again, but this time because the person has abandoned the patient. The staff is caught in a repetitive, no-win situation and, in essence, is trapped, as was the patient in the original abusive situation. In short, staff experience the abuse and are perplexed as to how to get out of it. They begin to overcompensate, trying to control their defensiveness and then pulling away or exploding at the patient, using the power of restrictions, medications, seclusion rooms, etc.

We are drawn to the patient's terror of reliving past horrifying hospital experiences; we are bombarded with challenges to power and authority and we are responsive to the experience of splitting between the 'good guys' and the 'bad guys.' And through all of this we are aware of feeling victimized, misunderstood, threatened, helpless, vindictive, and exhausted. These are parallel processes of the trauma experience of the patient. The trauma patient responds to the various providers as if they were the potential rescuer, healer of all, ally or exploiter, enemy, untrustworthy, and dangerous perpetrator. We cannot fail to respond. But how we respond is the therapeutic challenge.

Vicarious Traumatization 83

Even in knowing there is a trauma history, these shifts are stressful for the patient and the nurse because the immediate resolution of mistrust is not really possible. When patients challenge and threaten, such behavior invites a like response from the nurse. It takes time and patience to build enough trust for patients to experience feedback on their behavior as constructive and not feel insulted, manipulated, deceived, or betrayed. This is tedious work and is best done by a team approach to treatment and care. If the team can be open with one another, allow for differences, and realize what is going on, there is a better chance that the victim of violence can eventually reconnect without the defensive behaviors, experiencing the world of the team as not as unsafe as he/she fears. Victims of violence experience a total erosion of the possibility of a safe world of people, and the intense fear of and association with the past abuses of the trauma itself. The subsequent revictimization associated with the defensive behavior of the patient confronts the nurse with behaviors that are deeply entrenched. In turn, the nurse's sense of competency and effectiveness can be eroded, which can lead the nurse to either become overinvolved or to disengage. Either circumstance does not bode well for the nurse or for the nurse–patient relationship.

A final example underscores that as nurses we rarely enter into the struggles of victims of violence in a neutral manner. Institutional positions and societal myths regarding violence and victims permeate a nurse's response patterns and the positions taken with victims. In part this is because the multitude of systems involved with victims and perpetrators does not work together to protect and keep the focus. Rather, these systems are often adversarial and intimidating. The gist of the issues was the fact that in the process of a woman divorcing her abusive husband, she lost custody of the children because the abuse history could not be part of the evidence in the court handling custody. The mother had sought psychiatric help for the older child. The therapist seeing the child determined that the mother's anger toward the now ex-husband was so great that the children would not be able to develop a positive relationship with the father; therefore, the judge awarded custody to the father.

During the past month, the mother had the children for a summer vacation. During this time, the husband started legal actions against the mother, claiming that he had information that should limit the mother's visits with her children and that future visits should be supervised. The mother was now frantically trying to get an expert witness to enter into court the information on the battering to protect her rights with the children. According to the woman, however, the judge was not sympathetic to her requests for extra time to prepare for her defense. The woman's lawyer was not expert in the area of domestic abuse but was attempting to get a guardian *ad lidum* for the children. The woman indicated that she was in therapy. The nurse referred her to a specialized unit that dealt with domestic violence and had access to legal expertise specifically around these legal and evaluation issues.

84   *Nursing Care in a Violent Society: Issues and Research*

This last example shows how traumatic interpersonal violence can impact on a host of systems. In this case, the issue of domestic violence was addressed by various people in decision-making positions. The fragmented systems dealing with the issues of spousal abuse contribute to the confusion of the positions taken by professionals without a full picture of what has occurred. Over time, systems confusion engenders tremendous stress in providers, thus obliterating a sound, reasoned approach. Providers and service people become adversaries and replicate the family conflicts. Much of the conflict in this particular situation arose out of inadequate laws that allowed perpetrators of domestic violence to move from one court system, where the legal steps were executed to stop the violence against the wife, to another court system where issues of custody excluded past or ongoing issues related to spousal abuse from consideration in the matter of custody. While the law may change, the underlying problems have still not been addressed, and those are the biases held by providers and systems. When biases are addressed, there will be greater opportunities for an impartial review of parents' abilities to parent and of the impact of parenting assessed with regard to the children. In turn, professionals will not have the added burden of being adversaries.

When we are pulled into a situation where an ally is essential, we have crossed over therapeutic boundaries and must realize that this is at the risk of moving us toward Type II CTR responses. When we do this, it is important to have ongoing consultation, collaboration, and clarity as to what our role is in relation to the victim and the systems issues.

CONCLUSIONS

When nurses work with victims of violence, the traumatic events recounted by patients and witnessed by the nurse can result in the traumatization of the nurse. When victims of violence come to nurses for counseling, the defensive styles developed by nurses to deal with the symptoms and disruption of the patient's bio-behavioral systems pushes the limits of interpersonal tolerance. The style of presentation and the stress of the trauma story challenges the nurse's capacity to be empathic with the patient. The emotional arousal sets up a dynamic of approach and avoidance in the nurse–patient relationship. In turn, the dynamic is marked by Type I or Type II countertransference responses.

In either type, the nurse can expect deep reactions to the patient as patterns emerge in which nurses or patients can alter their roles and reactions toward the other, such as aggressor/agressee; exploiter/exploited; allies/enemies; rescuer/rescued. At times, the patient and nurse can be linked together in the roles with respect to a third party. This third party can be an institution, such as a hospital or other service agency or a third person, such as another care provider. A more destructive aspect in the nurse–patient relationship is when

Vicarious Traumatization

the hostility, fear, and anger are centered on the nurse as if the nurse is the perpetrator. It is as if the patient is reliving the violent event with the nurse. More subtle dimensions of reenactment occur when the patient places the nurse in an emotional bind that is similar to that of a patient and a perpetrator. Under these circumstances, the nurse may experience guilt, a deep sense of inadequacy, helplessness, and terror. In a more ominous vein, the patient may take revenge on the nurse for what happened. These distortions are not within the awareness of the patient, nor are they always amenable to interpretation.

The patient cannot respond in any other manner when threatened. It must be remembered that the signals for threat are not always within the awareness of the patient, nor is the patient, once threatened biologically and psychologically, sufficiently organized to alter a defensive reaction.

Noncompliance with health service recommendations, surly attitudes toward providers marked by distrust or, more perplexing, by appeals for help only to back off from efforts made on behalf of the patient, are but a few of the transactional pitfalls. Victims of violence, particularly those exploited and abused at an early age, look for splits in the relationships of those designated to provide care. These splits warn the patient not to trust. Expectations and demanding behavior countered by expectations and demanding behavior on the part of the nurse miss the inter- and intrapersonal structural processes that are linked to surviving the original violent abuses.

Nurses must take time out to reflect on the population of patients they work with, the impact of the trauma stories on them, and their own strong reactions to how they experience the patients engaging them. Consultation and case review are essential to maintain perspective and sustain an empathic stance necessary to help others. Personal care must be taken by nurses to ensure that their own lives include enrichment, support, and healthy living habits. Rest, exercise, and care with food and drink are basic. When these habits are combined with a review of the day-by-day response to work, a first step is taken by the individual nurse to prevent overload from the emotional demands of work with victims of violence.

Institutionally and professionally, policies and practices must be set up to help nurses in whatever setting they are in to deal with the stress of the emotional encounters they have with patients. Supervision, staff education, and consultation are not new concepts. In the cost-containment environment of the health care system, however, lack of attention to the work environment for nurses can result in higher costs in the long-run. The downsizing of hospitals and cuts in personnel and supportive programs for nurses in the direct care role mean that new and creative ways need to be developed to prevent the negative impact of working with traumatized patients. Within community-based programs, the potential for further isolation in matters of direct care will occur if practice policies and patterns are not established for a review and consultation for the many cases handled by individual nurse providers. Economic gain often comes

86   *Nursing Care in a Violent Society: Issues and Research*

by increasing the volume of contact at the expense of quality and consideration of the provider as well as the patient. To be able to listen and hear requires that those who are to listen can also be heard. When a system provides for this, the job of healing can proceed. Collective action must preserve the psychological health of nurses and the systems in which they work. Only in this way can effective and cost-conscious care can be provided.

REFERENCES

Buie, D. (June, 1994). *The hateful patient*. Paper presented at Bridgewater State Hospital, MA, Conference on Violence.

Caplan, G. (1970). *The theory and practice of mental health consultation*. New York: Basic Books.

Danieli, Y. (1980). Countertransference in the treatment and study of Nazi Holocaust survivors and their children. *Victimology: An International Journal, 5* (2-4), 355-367.

Danieli, Y. (1988). The use of mutual support approaches in the treatment of victims. In E. Chigier (Ed.), *Grief and bereavement in contemporary society. Support Systems, 3*,116-123.

Danieli, Y. (1985). The treatment and prevention of long-term effects and intergenerational transmission of vitimization: A lesson from Holocaust survivors and their children. In C.R. Figley (Ed.), *Trauma and its wake* (pp. 15-35). New York: Brunner/Mazel.

Eth, S., & Pynoos, R. S. (1985). *Post-traumatic stress disorder in children*. Washington DC: American Psychiatric Press.

Figley, C. R. (1988). A five-phase treatment of post traumatic stress disorder in families. *Journal of Traumatic Stress, 1* (1), 127-141.

Figley, C. R. (Ed.). (In press). *Compassion fatigue: Secondary traumatic stress disorder from treating the traumatized*. New York: Brunner/Mazel.

Friedman, M. J. (1993). Psychobiological and pharmacological approaches to treatment. In J. P. Wilson & B. Raphael (Eds.), *International handbook of traumatic stress syndrome* (pp. 785–794). New York: Plenum Press.

Giller, E. (1990) (Ed.). Biological assessment and treatment of posttraumatic stress disorder. In *Progress in psychiatry series*. Washington, DC: American Psychiatric Press, Inc.

Gleser, G. C., Green, B. L., & Winget, C. (1981). *Prolonged psychological effects of Disaster: A study of Buffalo Creek*. New York: Academic Press.

Haley, S. A. (1974). When a patient reports atrocities: Specific treatment considerations in the Vietnam veteran. *Archives of General Psychiatry, 30,* 191-196.

Hartman, C. R., & Burgess, A. W. (1988). Information of trauma: A case application of the model. *Journal of Interpersonal Violence, 3*(4), 443-457.

Hartman, C. R., & Burgess, A. G., Burgess, A. W., & Kelley, S. J. (1992). Extrafamilial child sexual abuse: Family-focused intervention. In A. W. Burgess (Ed.), *Child trauma I: Issues & Research* (pp. 307-334). New York: Garland Publishing.

Hartman, C. R., & Burgess, A. W. (1993). Information processing of trauma. *Child Abuse and Neglect, 17* (1), 47-58.

Hartman, C. R., & Jackson, H. (1994). Rape and the phenomena of countertransference. In J. P. Wilson & J. D. Lindy (Eds.), *Countertransference in the treatment of PTSD* (pp. 206-244). New York: Guilford Press.

Vicarious Traumatization

Hartsough, D. M. (1988). Traumatic stress as an area for research. *Journal of Traumatic Stress*, *1*(2), 145 -154.

Herman, J. W. (1992). *Trauma and recovery*. New York: Basic Books.

Hinshaw, A. S., & Atwood, J. R. (1984). Nursing staff turnover, stress, and satisfaction: Models, measures, and management. In H. H. Werley & J. J. Fitzpatrick (Eds.), *Annual review of nursing research* (Vol. 2, pp. 133-153). New York: Springer Publishing Co.

Horowitz, M. (1976). Intrusive and repetitive thoughts after experimental stress. *Archives of General Psychiatry*, *32*, 1457-1463.

Jacobson, S. F., & McGrath, H. M. (1983). *Nurses under stress*. New York: John Wiley & Sons.

Kelley, S. J. (1992). Stress responses of children and parents to sexual abuse and ritualistic abuse in day care centers. In A. W. Burgess (Ed.), *Child trauma 1: Issues & research* (pp. 231-258). New York: Garland Publishing.

Kluft, R. P. (1989). The rehabilitation of therapists overwhelmed by their work with multiple personality disorder patients. *Dissociation*, *2*, 244-250.

Kluft, R. P. (1994). Countertransference in the treatment of multiple personality disorder. In J.P. Wilson & J. D. Lindy (Eds.), *Countertransference in the treatment of PTSD*, (pp. 122 -150). New York: Guilford Press.

Langer, R. (1987). Post-traumatic stress disorder in former POWS. In T. Williams (Ed.). *Post-traumatic stress disorders: A handbook for clinicians* (pp. 35-50). *Disabled American Veterans*. Cincinnati, OH.

Livingston, M., & Livingston, H. (1984). Emotional distress in nurses at work. *British Journal of Medical Psychology*, *57*, 291-294.

McCann, I. L., & Pearlman, L. A. (1990). *Psychological trauma and the adult survivor*. New York: Brunner/Mazel.

McEwen, B. S., & Mendelson, S. (1993). Effects of stress on the neurochemistry and morphology of the brain: Counterregulation versus damage. In L. Godberger & S. Breznets (Eds.), *Handbook of stress: Theoretical and clinical aspects* (2nd Ed., pp. 101-126). New York: Free Press.

Monica, R. F. (1988). The trauma story: The psychiatric care of refugee survivors of violence and torture. In F. M. Ochberg (Ed.), *Post-traumatic therapy and victims of violence* (pp. 295-314). New York: Brunner/Mazel.

Munroe, J. F. (1991). *Therapist traumatization from exposure to clients with combat-related post-traumatic stress disorder: Implications for administration and supervision.* Unpublished doctoral dissertation, available from Dissertation Abstracts, Ann Arbor, Michigan.

Munroe, J. F., Shay J., Fisher, L., Makary, C., Rapperport, K., & Zimering, R. (June, 1994). *Trauma Group Meeting.* Presentation of research and team work in the management of stress in the provider.

Norbeck, J. S. (1986). Perceived job stress, job satisfaction, and psychological symptoms in critical care nursing. *Research in Nursing and Health*, *34*(4) 225-230.

Putnam, F. W. (1989). *Diagnosis and treatment of multiple personality disorder*. New York: Guilford Press.

Pynoos, R. S.,& Nader, K. (1988). Psychological first aid and treatment approach to children exposed to community violence: Research implications. *Journal of Traumatic Stress*, *1*(4), 445-474.

Racker, H. (1968). *Transference and Countertransference*. New York: International Universities Press.

Slatker, E. (1987). *Countertransference*. New York: Jason Aronson.

Solomon, Z. (1990). *From front line to home front: Wives of PTSD veterans*. Paper presented at the sixth annual meeting of the Society for Traumatic Stress Studies, New Orleans, LA.

Stanton, A. H., & Schwartz, M. S. (1954). *The mental hospital.* New York: Basic Books.

Sullivan, H. S. (1953) *The interpersonal theory of psychiatry.* New York: W. W. Norton & Company, Inc.

Utterback, J., & Caldwell, J. (1989.) Proactive and reactive approaches to PTSD in the aftermath of campus violence: Forming a traumatic stress reaction team. *Journal of Traumatic Stress, 2*(2), 153-169.

Vachon, M. L. S. (1987). *Occupational stress in the care of the critically ill, the dying and the bereaved.* New York: Hemisphere Publishing Corporation.

Van der Kolk, B. A., & Saporta, J. (1993). Biological response to psychic trauma. In J. P. Wilson & B. Raphael (Eds.), *International handbook of traumatic stress syndromes* (pp. 25-33). New York: Plenum Press.

Wilson, J. P. (1989). *Trauma, transformation and healing—An interactive approach to theory, research, and post traumatic therapy.* New York: Brunner/Mazel.

Wilson, J. P., & Lindy, J. D. (1994). *Countertransference in the treatment of PTSD.* New York: Guilford Press.

6

Ethical Problems in Caring for Violent Psychiatric Patients

Anastasia Fisher

Psychiatric nursing practice in acute inpatient and emergency settings requires that practitioners identify and manage dangerous patients. The analyses reported here are part of a broader study that sought to understand how psychiatric nurses define and manage the dangerous mentally ill. This chapter identifies three ethical problems encountered in the day-to-day practices of psychiatric nurses, as they cared for and managed the dangerous mentally ill. The three ethical problems, balancing support for patient autonomy with the need to maintain unit control; balancing the need for distancing with the desire to establish therapeutic relationships; and balancing the desire to "do the right thing" with the need to get along with colleagues, have implications for psychiatric nursing practice and the institutional settings that treat the dangerous mentally ill. Additionally, this study provides direction for further inquiry into the actual ethical problems encountered in practice.

Dangerousness represents the single most significant criterion justifying both involuntary commitment of the mentally ill and emergency interventions within psychiatric treatment settings (Cocozza & Steadman, 1977; Monahan, 1984). Psychiatric nursing practice in acute inpatient and emergency settings requires that practitioners identify and manage dangerous patients. Historically, psychiatric nurses have assumed responsibility for creating and maintaining safe environments for patients and staff (Cahill, Stuart, Laraia, & Arana, 1991; Sclafani, 1986). This tradition, requiring that staff act quickly to predict and control potential violence, remains a significant component of contemporary nursing work in psychiatric emergency and inpatient settings (Anderson & Roper, 1991; Grey & Diers, 1992; Morrison, 1993). The increased public attention to the incidence of interpersonal violence in society (Rigdon, 1994), coupled with the evidence of escalating violence within hospitals (Davis, 1991; Snyder, 1994), magnifies the importance of understanding psychiatric nursing practice with the dangerous mentally ill.

While it is generally agreed that it is morally acceptable and professionally justifiable to restrict an individual's liberty when that person's liberty could cause harm to others, it is also recognized that interventions to control behavior in psychiatric settings require justification (Beauchamp & Childress, 1989;

89

Davis & Aroskar, 1991; Gaylin, 1974; Kittrie, 1971; Sclafani, 1986). On first glance these responsibilities, actions, and justifications may seem rather straightforward but, in fact, there are genuine ethical problems associated with dangerousness and its management.

Before moving into a discussion of the ethical problems associated with dangerousness, it may be helpful to point out some of the problems with the terminology *dangerous mentally ill,* as it is generally recognized that dangerousness is an ambiguous term without an accepted meaning (Shah, 1977, 1978). Dangerousness refers to the prediction of future violence. In the case of this study, the prediction is being applied to mentally ill persons. This estimation of the potential that a person will do something in the future that is defined as dangerous is based on the perception that a person possessing certain characteristics or demonstrating certain behaviors has a higher probability of performing certain acts in the future than someone who doesn't have the characteristics or who doesn't engage in the behavior (Steadman, 1980). Brooks (1978) suggested that this lack of a shared meaning about what constitutes dangerousness results in practitioners providing their own personal subjective definitions. These subjective definitions have tended to reflect the individual idiosyncratic values of the clinicians and the various political pressures they experience. Among the public, this lack of clarity in terminology contributes to assumptions that most individuals who commit a violent act are mentally ill and that most mentally ill individuals are dangerous (Cocozza & Steadman, 1977). It is not the position here, however, that all mentally ill persons are dangerous. On the contrary, it is suggested that dangerousness, rather than being a characteristic or attribute of individuals, is constructed and defined contextually and is to some extent, as with beauty, "in the eye of the beholder" (Fisher, 1989; Stone, 1976). This ambiguity, no doubt, contributes to the ethical problems inherent in defining, labeling, and managing those mentally ill individuals who are dangerous.

Since defining persons as dangerous can restrict their liberty in the absence of actual violent behavior and rationalize the restriction on the basis of the well-being of others and of the individual, how nurses make decisions about dangerous patients and how they manage their behavior, are therefore, important practice issues. Davis & Aroskar (1991) suggest that this is the basic ethical problem of behavior control. There has been much attention paid in the bioethical, medico-legal, and nursing literature to topics relevant to patient danger and its management. Among the relevant topics are concepts: autonomy, beneficence, coercion, and social and behavior control (Cocozza & Steadman, 1977; Davis, 1978; Dworkin, 1978; Garritson-Hunn, 1983; Garritson-Hunn & Davis, 1983; Gaylin, 1974; Halleck, 1974; London, 1977; McCloskey, 1980; Outlaw & Lowery, 1992; Steadman, 1972; Stilling, 1992; Stone, 1975; Tardiff, 1984). Ethical research in psychiatric nursing practice is, however, more limited (Carpenter, 1991; Forchuk, 1991; Garritson-Hunn, 1988;

Ethical Problems   91

Liaschenko, 1993; Lützén, 1990; Lützén & Nordin, 1993) and does not focus specifically on work with the dangerous mentally ill.

Ethics research in psychiatric nursing reveals a variety of philosophical and methodological approaches to inquiry and demonstrates variations in findings. Among the philosophical approaches used to guide this research are the principle-based approach, an ethic of care, and a practice-based morality. The principle-based approach to ethics relies on rules and principles to guide and justify our ethical choices. Important concepts within this approach are rights, duty, obligation, justice, and autonomy (Davis & Aroskar, 1991). This approach is well represented in the medical and nursing ethics literature and is "considered to represent the dominant conception of morality in this country" (Cooper, 1990, p. 210). The ethics of care began with the work of Leininger (1977) and Watson (1979) and makes care central to nursing practice. The last approach in the ethics literature is a practice account of morality and is based on the notion that "practice has embedded within it a morality derived from the activities of that practice" (Liaschenko, 1993, p. vii). Practices are collective human activities that meet a social need, such as caring for children, caring for the sick, protecting the citizenry, etc. (Liaschenko, 1993; Ruddick, 1989). In this approach, ethical considerations are internal to practice rather than a series of rules located apart from situations that then must be applied to practice. In her 1993 narrative examination of psychiatric and community health nurses, Liaschenko identified "helping patients to have a life" as the essential moral dimension in practice. Liaschenko (1993) questions the philosophical traditions of a principle-based ethic and the emerging perspective of an "ethic of care" that have provided the foundational frameworks in previous ethics research, and proposes, instead, a practice conception of morality.

Although the psychiatric nursing ethics literature has used these different philosophical approaches, several studies have identified beneficence or "doing good" and the need to balance beneficence with autonomy as the most significant moral concept related to psychiatric nurses' decision making (Forchuk, 1991; Garritson, 1988; Lützén & Nordin, 1993). Tentative findings from the studies by Carpenter (1991) and Forchuk (1991) identified ethical decision making and staff conflict as contributing to stress among inpatient nurses, which may result in their choice to leave the profession. Each of these studies contributes to further understanding of the ethical dimensions in psychiatric nursing work and invites further inquiry and debate into the ethical nature of practice.

The analyses reported here are part of a broader study that sought to understand how psychiatric nurses define and manage acutely ill psychiatric inpatients who are dangerous toward patients, staff, family, and strangers. For this investigation, the term "dangerousness" was limited to the perception and prediction that a person will demonstrate assaultive or violent behavior toward others. Notable among the findings from that broader work were the extent of

92   *Nursing Care in a Violent Society: Issues and Research*

disagreement among subjects regarding what consitutes danger toward others in this patient population and the influence of context (staffing, number of admissions, census, etc.) on defining and managing danger. In the course of discussing their work, psychiatric nurses talked about the moral problems arising from actions they had taken toward patients. These actions led them to question the kind of persons they are, their relationships with colleagues, and their practice.

This chapter describes those ethical problems encountered by psychiatric nurses in their practice with the dangerous mentally ill. They are representative of the ethical problems found in the day-to-day practices of psychiatric nurses. What is striking about these findings is their emergence in a study about practice, and not about ethics. This discovery supports an approach to ethics that acknowledges that practice has a morality embedded within it that deserves to be explored and explicated. The purposes of this chapter are to provide an understanding of an aspect of contemporary psychiatric nursing work with the dangerous mentally ill and to give nurses a language for the actual ethical problems they encounter in their practice (Holly, 1993; Liaschenko, 1993). In so doing, this report shifts attention away from the principle-based accounts of bioethics to those of specific practices and goals that are embedded in context, experience, and relationship (Cooper, 1990; Liaschenko, 1993; Lützén & Nordin, 1993).

METHODOLOGY

Setting

For this study, data were collected from psychiatric nursing personnel who practiced on two locked inpatient units in a large urban medical center. The two units, a locked civil commitment unit and a maximum security forensic unit, were chosen for their diversity in structure, control, and treatment philosophy because these conditions were thought to influence nurses' decision making about patient danger and the actions nurses would take in response. Use of these units permitted exploration of their differences in order to understand the influence of contextual conditions on nursing practice in relation to decisions about patient danger.

The ongoing census of the locked civil commitment unit was 21 functionally impaired and impoverished chronic mentally ill persons. During the conduct of this research, nearly 97% of the patients were admitted to the unit involuntarily, either as an emergency admission or on a conservatorship. Conservatorship appointments are made on the basis of persons' inability to provide for their basic needs, rather than on the basis of dangerousness, and require a judicial review. Appointments are renewable yearly. The other

Ethical Problems 93

approximately 3% of the patient population were voluntary admissions (2.4%) or their legal status on admission could not be determined from the chart review (1.2%). The unit was composed of two treatment teams: one emphasized a culturally sensitive program designed to meet the special mental health needs of the Latino population, and the other stressed the special mental health needs of women.

The forensic security unit served 12 patients and functioned as an inpatient extension for the city jail system by addressing the acute psychiatric needs of persons with serious criminal charges. All of these patients were admitted involuntarily on a 72-hour emergency hold or on a conservatorship.

Sample

The sample consisted of 18 members of the nursing staff, including registered nurses (70%), licensed psychiatric technicians (23%), and orderlies (7%) recruited from the two units described above. The sample was predominantly Caucasian, female, and 30 to 50 years of age, and had been employed full-time from 1 to 3 years at this institution. The study received approval from the Institutional Review Board, and all subjects gave signed consent prior to participating in the study.

Design

A field design was used in order to study practice as close to actual clinical situations as possible. Participant observation was conducted on the two units and field notes were recorded and later transcribed. During periods of observation, staff were engaged in informal conversations about what they were thinking and doing as they cared for patients.

Semi-structured interviews were conducted both at the institution and away from the work situation, depending upon each subject's preference. During the interviews, which varied in length from 1 to 3 hours, each subject was asked a series of open-ended questions to elicit background work and education history. These initial questions were followed by more specific probing: "How do you characterize problematic patient situations?" "What kinds of situations pose a danger to you, the unit, other staff?" "How are disagreements about these worked out among staff?" "How are agreements and disagreements about what constitutes danger communicated among staff?" A final series of questions was designed to elicit specific information from subjects about their patient management decisions, about changes they had noted in their practice over the years, and about their history of being assaulted or witnessing assaults at work. As mentioned previously, subjects were not asked specific questions about the ethical problems they encountered in practice. Interviews were conducted over a 1-year period, and were audiotaped and transcribed for subsequent analysis.

Analysis

The techniques of constant comparative analysis and dimensional analysis from the grounded theory method were utilized to analyze the data (Bowers, 1984; Fisher, 1989; Glaser & Strauss, 1967; Glaser, 1978; Hatton, 1985; Olshansky, 1985; Schatzman, 1991; Strauss, 1987). In keeping with the grounded theory method, data collection and analysis occurred simultaneously, rather than as two distinct phases.

Although the analytic stages are described here in a stepwise fashion for purposes of clarity, they actually occurred as an interactive process: Transcripts were reviewed generally for initial impressions and to obtain a broad sense of meaning, and data that related to the phenomenon of interest were identified. These data were coded as dimensions and further subdimensionalized into aspects or properties of the phenomenon. Memos were written related to initial hunches and questions, and tentative definitions were given to the initial dimensions and subdimensions. Each transcript was then further explored to identify the conditions, context, action, and consequences associated with each dimension and subdimension. Additional memos were written to describe emerging relationships among the dimensions and subdimensions. The salient dimensions and subdimensions, conditions, context, action, and consequences were then organized from the perspective of professional nurses at work into a matrix of considerations. Diagrams of the emerging schema were developed. The evolving description was validated with subjects throughout the analysis and data collection procedures.

FINDINGS

The analysis revealed three ethical problems encountered in psychiatric nursing practice with the dangerous mentally ill. These were: (a) *balancing support for patient autonomy with the need to maintain unit control,* (b) *balancing the need for distancing with the desire to establish therapeutic relationships,* and (c) *balancing the desire to "do the right thing" with the need to get along with colleagues.*

Balancing Support for Patient Autonomy with the Need to Maintain Control

Balancing support for patient autonomy with the need to maintain unit control was experienced by subjects as a tension between their desire to give patients latitude to manage their own behaviors and their simultaneous responsibility for maintaining unit safety. As one subject described it, this balancing is the essence of psychiatric nursing practice: "...my whole job is to balance how

Ethical Problems

much control to allow the patient and how much control to assume." In the example that follows, a subject anguishes over the decision to give a patient the opportunity to manage his own behavior:

> I thought we were beginning to develop a good trusting relationship, but this particular day I got a funny feeling from what he was saying. He managed to contain his anger, but then walked into the dining room and hit another patient. He drew blood. I felt like I should have been able to see that coming. I wanted to give him a chance because he had handled himself before.

Another subject stated, "I'm always asking myself, 'Did I act punitively?' 'Did his [the patient's] actions warrant my reaction?' or 'Did I act too quickly?'" These data characterize the actual mental struggle of the psychiatric nurses as they attempted to find this balance in their practice. Learning to *balance support for patient autonomy with the need to maintain unit control* evolved with experience in practice. Below two nurses discuss having to learn to establish control:

> My tendency initially was to intervene too late because I wanted to give the patient the benefit of the doubt. It's better to prevent something from happening. Now, I intervene early to take away some [patient] control, and give it back gradually.

> As my experience and fear of being injured grew, I would take a more controlling stance. I take all the power away from patients and give it back when they can handle it.

Although these examples demonstrate the subjects' struggle to *balance patient autonomy with maintenance of unit control,* they often came down on the side of control. Coming down on the side of control means that subjects often intervened early to contain patients, thus limiting the patients' opportunity to manage their own behavior in less restrictive ways. This emphasis on the need to maintain unit control, and thus a safe environment, resulted in the early implementation of control-oriented interventions. More controlling interventions, such as medicating, or secluding and restraining, were chosen rather than short time-outs (retreat from the stimulating environment for 5 to 10 minutes) or talking to patients. Often, these strategies were initiated in a routinized manner without regard for the condition of the patient. Subjects came down on the side of control because they believed they were in jeopardy from the patients and that control was the best way to achieve safety. Examples follow:

> I'm always concerned about my own safety. That is the bottom line, the safety of the patients, the other staff, and myself. Safety is my bottom line—the most important thing.

> To me, safety is the top priority when I go into a psychiatric setting, not the quality of my therapeutic interaction. That is on my agenda, but it's not my top priority.

I'm looking to save me. The only consideration is the physical harm intervening will create for me. I don't want to get hurt.

In addition, subjects came down on the side of unit control because they'd learned it was a priority to their coworkers. Staff experienced significant pressure from colleagues to conform their practice to the standards and treatment philosophy of the unit. For many subjects, this meant relinquishing their values about professional conduct toward patients for those of the dominant group culture. As one nurse said:

When I first started in psychiatry, I had a humanistic view of dealing with patients. I was under the impression that by talking to patients, at some point, I'd reach them. But that wasn't the way at [this hospital]. Right away, staff made it clear to me they were not ready to spend a lot of time talking to patients. I was told, "If patients don't respond to a request right away, we grab 'em and do whatever we have to." It was punishment.

The degree of *balancing support for patient autonomy with the need to maintain unit control* that was required by subjects was influenced by the contextual considerations of individual and collective tolerances. Tolerances refer to the willingness "to put up with" particular patient behaviors, attributes or work conditions. Personal tolerances were those held by individual members of staff. Collective tolerance was established by the unit's treatment philosophy or the "rules of the game" on the unit, and thus was contextual. It is important to note that the individual tolerance of a staff person was modified by the collective tolerance of the unit. As subjects on the jail unit noted:

It's important for the staff to be consistent. Everyone has to observe the rules. If a patient comes to you and calls you a b— and you do nothing and then he says the same thing to another nurse and gets put into seclusion, everything breaks down. You have to forget your tolerance and go with the rule on the unit.

We are more strict on the jail unit. Patients have to take medications. We offer it once, if they don't take it, we put them down and give an injection. There is less negotiation.

Of the two units included in this study, the jail unit was particularly focused on safety and control, and had clearer behavioral expectations for both patient and staff. Although nurses experienced the unit as safer than other settings within the department, they acknowledged the general intolerance for autonomous decision making among the nursing staff. Here the unit expectations and rules were clear, non-negotiable, readily implemented, and organized around safety considerations, thus reducing the need to *balance support for patient autonomy with maintenance of unit control.* As we saw in the preceding examples, by relying on the rules of the unit, subjects were required to use little discretionary judgment. This first problem emphasized the subjects' concern for unit safety while the next, *balancing the need for distance with the desire to establish therapeutic relationships,* examines the subjects' concern for their personal safety.

Ethical Problems

Balancing the Need for Distance with the Desire to Establish Therapeutic Relationships

Balancing the need for distance with the desire to establish therapeutic relationships was experienced by subjects as a tension between the construction and maintenance of emotional and physical separation from patients and their desire for a therapeutic alliance with patients. On the one hand, subjects desired knowing the patient through an interpersonal relationship; on the other hand, they were concerned for their personal safety, which interfered with their establishing a relationship with the patient. This desire, yet inability to establish therapeutic relationships with patients, contributed to subjects' maintaining their perspective of patients as dangerous and reinforced their belief that patients must be kept at a distance. Distancing operated as a strategy to protect subjects from physical assault, maintain their sense of safety, maintain their image as professionals, and manage their fears. Its use, however, left subjects conflicted about their practice and their professional responsibilities toward patients. This, in turn, created long-term, often unresolved, guilt, shame, and grief in relation to their professional identity and responsibilities. Examples from the data follow:

> I don't let these patients get physically close to me. I never turn my back on them, touch them, or share small talk with them, and of course they don't touch me."

> I am aloof toward the patients. It causes me some degree of guilt and grief. I think maybe I don't interact enough or give them enough.

In spite of their concern for safety and need for distance, some subjects were able to transcend their sense of danger. One described this process poignantly:

> I look for something I can relate to, something that will allow us to relate to one another. Our sameness. If I never get close to them [the patients], I can't discover these things. Once I find the sameness, I am more likely to find something I like. Then, they seem less dangerous.

This ethical problem raises significant issues regarding relationships between nurses and patients. It also raises important questions about the nature of that relationship within acute psychiatric institutions and points out the work required, by subjects, to establish a connection with these patients.

Balancing Wanting to "Do the Right Thing" With the Need to Get Along With Colleagues

The final ethical problem identified was *balancing wanting to "do the right thing" with the need to get along with colleagues.* This problem was experienced by subjects as a tension between their desire to do what was right for a patient and their desire to get along with their colleagues. They often found that to do what was right for their patients put them in conflict with coworkers, supervisors, and administrators. *Doing the right thing* referred to decisions and actions that were made with the patients' best interests as central. Decisions and actions that were made with the patients' best interest as central often involved tolerating some disturbing or annoying behaviors while the patient tried to manage them, rather than the staff immediately initiating restrictive interventions to contain these problematic behaviors. Initiating interventions always involved judgments and decisions about patient care for which there were a variety of possibilities. When staff, in an effort to do the right thing, made decisions and initiated interventions that were less control-oriented (such as watching or talking rather than medicating or secluding), they were often defined by coworkers as inexperienced, as victims of manipulation, or as not acting as a team member. When this occurred, doing the right thing was in conflict with getting along with colleagues. The following examples identify the pressure on staff to conform their practice to that of the dominant group culture in order to get along with their colleagues:

> After awhile, I stopped worrying about punishing interventions toward patients, and I worried about my own safety. I wanted to get along with the people I worked with; I wanted to fit in, no matter how uncomfortable it was for me inside; I wanted to be part of the group; I just went along with it.

> I did something that was really against my better judgment. I was stupid. I wanted to wait and see, but...[the charge nurse] made me feel that I wasn't doing my job.

> I don't want to separate myself from the group. I depend on them, when violent situations come up, I need to know that these people will come and help me.

Although subjects wanted to do the right thing, getting along with colleagues took precedence. *Getting along with colleagues* took precedence because staff depended on one another to manage violent situations. As one subject recalled, "...there was always a nagging worry in the back of my mind that she'd [a colleague] leave me hanging out in the wind again." Disagreements about patient behavior, the level of danger it posed, and how to manage it placed staff relationships, and thus one's physical safety, in jeopardy. Staff members indicated that by challenging the group norms for defining and managing patient behaviors, they risked losing their colleagues' support in emergency situations and being left alone to manage a dangerous patient. When wanting to do the right thing conflicted with getting along with colleagues, and it often did, subjects experienced an increased sense of vulnerability and risk regarding both their personal safety and their image of themselves as nurses.

Doing the right thing for patients sometimes involved dealing with issues of abusive behaviors by colleagues. As a subject indicated, "It isn't always the patient who is dangerous." Or as another subject noted, "I'm talking about staff who create situations, knowingly or unknowingly, that intimidate patients and

Ethical Problems

that end violently." These observations about problematic staff behaviors were, for the most part, privately held, as this was a topic that deeply saddened and threatened the subjects. One subject shared this painful account, "This issue [of staff abuse toward patients] rarely comes up. We don't know how to talk about it with each other. It's easier to ignore it." Some subjects noted that they had tried to *do the right thing* by going to the administration with their observations about abusive staff behaviors, but had found the institutional response itself harsh and punitive. These harsh institutional responses contributed to subjects' guilt for trying to *do the right thing* and discouraged them from trying to intervene in future episodes. As one subject stated:

> Institutions are not as well set up to deal with abusive staff as they are to deal with violent patients. Administration usually ends up eliminating the staff member after things go too far. We set up staff members for mistreatment from their colleagues rather than deal with them professionally.

The interaction of abusive staff behaviors with abusive institutional responses appeared to contribute to the secretive nature of staff abuse toward patients. This further perpetuated incidents and increased the difficulties for patients, staff, and administrators to deal effectively with this significant practice issue. The tension between wanting to do the right thing and the need to get along with colleagues raises some interesting questions about practice and the culture of our work environments. For example: "In what types of environments can doing the right thing and getting along coexist?"; "Is there something unique about working with the dangerous mentally ill that supports or magnifies this tension?"; and "What clinical and institutional strategies can be implemented to reduce this tension?" It is apparent from the powerful examples shared by the subjects that the tension between wanting to do the right thing and the need to get along with colleagues had significance for the staff, patients, and institutions. As one subject noted, "I left work because I couldn't tolerate the staff's brutality toward the patients and what it was doing to me. I couldn't stand the pressure."

DISCUSSION

Three ethical problems, balancing support for patient autonomy with the need to maintain unit control; balancing the need for distancing with the desire to establish therapeutic relationships; and balancing the desire to do the right thing with the need to get along with colleagues, were identified in a study of contemporary psychiatric nursing practice. This particular practice is organized around the provision of care to dangerous mentally ill persons and the requirement to maintain safety. While all subjects in this study identified these problems and acknowledged the accuracy of this representation of their practice, it is premature to conclude that these problems are inherent in all nursing practice, or even in all psychiatric nursing practice. It is likely, however, that these problems may be present to some degree in all nursing practice situations, as a number of other studies (Forchuk, 1991; Garritson, 1988; Jenks, 1993; Lützén & Nordin, 1993) have either hinted at or clearly identified similar ethical issues as central to practice. Further research that seeks to understand the nature of the ethical considerations encountered in nursing practice will be required before attempting to generalize this work to other settings and situations.

Findings presented in this chapter clearly reflect the impact of the organizational context on the behavior of psychiatric nurses, yet few details have been provided about the patients. They deserve, however, to be represented in this examination, for without them there would be no practice. Because of the vulnerability of these patients and our wish not to further their suffering, it is easy to neglect the fact that these patients are often threatening, intimidating, rejecting, and physically repulsive to their caregivers. Sometimes they are violent toward their caregivers and toward other patients for whom these caregivers are also responsible. Because it is easy to neglect acknowledging these negative patient characteristics, it is also easy to forget that these patients present legitimate concerns to the nurses who care for them and who must manage their behavior. Results from this study have implications for institutions, practitioners, and administrators as they work to create more humane environments in an era of mental health care reform and cost-containment.

The findings organize themselves around the nature of relationships in psychiatric nursing practice. Repeatedly the subjects in this study struggled in their relationships with patients and with coworkers. These relationships were situated in institutional settings where nursing staff cared for and managed dangerous mentally ill patients. Perhaps the need to wonder about the nature of these relationships in contemporary psychiatric nursing work is long overdue. The original emphasis on the nurse–patient relationship grew out of an era in psychiatric care when the psychological paradigm was dominant. That paradigm was characterized by long-term treatment and the centrality of relationship and largely ignored the biological basis of illness (Liaschenko, 1989). Today's realities are very different in acute inpatient and emergency psychiatric settings, reflecting problems of the larger society. Contemporary mental health policies emphasize brief, involuntary hospitalizations for the most dangerous of the mentally ill, as well as psychopharmacological interventions, downsizing, and increased use of nonprofessionals as careproviders.

Given the nature of the current practice environment, and the findings from the study reported here, a number of relevant questions can be raised. Among them are: What is the nature of relationship in psychiatric nursing practice with patients who are frightening and dangerous as well as severely mentally ill? How are we to educate nurses to practice psychiatric nursing in environments

Ethical Problems 101

that care for the dangerous mentally ill? How are nurses to practice in an environment emphasizing control over relationship? Can the emphasis on control be changed? What kind of practice is possible in such an environment? How can administrators reorganize care to accommodate relationship? If nurses can build bridges between themselves and unlikeable patients in an effort to make a connection, as Liaschenko (1994) has suggested, we must wonder how this work (of building bridges) is to be accomplished with the dangerous mentally ill. Findings from this study only hint at the work required of nurses to build bridges to their dangerous mentally ill patients. Given Heifner's (1993) findings that even in the presence of "connectedness" nurses maintain distance from patients, the nature of the nurse–patient relationship in psychiatric nursing is an area worthy of our attention.

In addition to the nurse–patient relationship, subjects in this study also struggled in their relationships with coworkers. Findings suggest that the subjects entered practice invested in the individual patient. They came to practice with a genuine desire to do their best for their patients, to help them, care for them, and remain compassionate toward them. Once in practice, however, they found these values impossible to maintain. They felt pressure from their colleagues to conform their practice and they soon learned that to work in this kind of institutional setting required compromising those values. This compromise resulted in use of overcontrolling interventions with patients. A study of knowing in decision making revealed similar findings from a psychiatric nurse (Jenks, 1993). In that study, too, the psychiatric nurse responded to pressure from coworkers, deviating from her beliefs and changing her practice. Her changed practice involved giving a patient medications rather than letting things unfold, as had been her original decision. Jenks suggested that it was the most experienced nurses who felt the need to preserve their relationships with staff, while less experienced nurses needed to establish colleagial relationships. Jenks's findings, coupled with those from the current study, are troubling and lead one to wonder about the nature of the psychiatric nurse's relationship with colleagues. Among the questions raised are: What about psychiatric nursing practice requires this level of conformity? When is it acceptable to subjugate one's values about practice and one's clinical judgment to the will of one's coworkers? What are the long-term consequences of this submission for the nurse and the practice? How can institutions intervene in this process? It is particularly important that we attempt to answer these questions, given the evidence that controlling, coercive interactions with patients contribute to violence (Morrison, 1990, 1992). Efforts to reduce violent incidents in hospital settings will require moving our practice in the direction of increased cooperation and negotiation among staff and patients (Johnson & Morrison, 1993).

These struggles in relationship have occurred in specific institutional contexts. While it has long been appreciated that institutions are powerful,

102   *Nursing Care in a Violent Society: Issues and Research*

coercive, and regimented environments for patients, less attention has been given to the effect of these environments on nursing practice (Goffman, 1961). This lack of attention to the environment limits nursing's ability to understand its practice and limits the options for changing practice. Findings from this study indicate the important role of context on practice. It is clear in this work that unit context and institutional culture influenced nurses' behavior control practices, as has been suggested previously by Morrison (1990).

Finally, the ethical problems identified and the questions raised in this chapter are important to consider, given the current trend of admitting increasingly violent patients to acute psychiatric facilities. If more humane environments are to be created for practitioners and patients (Strumpf & Tomes, 1993), it has to be recognized that the care of dangerous persons has serious implications for psychiatric nurses, their work, and the institutions where they practice.

REFERENCES

Anderson, N. L. R., & Roper, J. M. (1991). The interactional dynamics of violence, Part II: Juvenile detention. *Archives of Psychiatric Nursing, 5,* 216-222.

Beauchamp, T. L., & Childress, J. F. (1989). *Principles of biomedical ethics.* New York: Oxford University Press.

Bowers, B. J. (1984). *Intergeneration care taking: Processes and consequences of creating knowledge.* Unpublished doctoral dissertation, University of California, San Francisco.

Brooks, A. D. (1978). Notes on defining dangerousness of the mentally ill. In C. J. Fredericks (Ed.), *Dangerous behavior: A problem in law and mental health.* (DHEW Publication No. ADM 78-563, pp. 37-60). Washington, DC: U.S. Government Printing Office.

Cahill, C. D., Stuart, G. W., Laraia, M. T., & Arana, G. W. (1991). Inpatient management of violent behavior: Nursing prevention and intervention. *Issues in Mental Health Nursing, 12,* 239-252.

Carpenter, M. A. (1991). The process of ethical decision making in psychiatric nursing practice. *Issues in Mental Health Nursing, 12,* 179-191.

Cocozza, J. J., & Steadman, H. J. (1977). Dangerousness and the social control of the mentally ill. In P. Wickman (Ed.), *Contemporary perspectives in social problems* (pp. 242-246). New York: HarperRow.

Cooper, M. C. (1990). Reconceptualizing nursing ethics. *Scholarly Inquiry for Nursing Practice: An International Journal, 4,* 209-222.

Davis, A. J. (1978). The ethics of behavior control: The nurse as double agent. *Issues in Mental Health Nursing, 1,* 2-16.

Davis, A. J., & Aroskar, M. A. (1991). *Ethical dilemmas and nursing practice.* Connecticut: Appleton & Lange.

Davis, S. (1991). Violence by psychiatric inpatients: A review. *Hospital & Community Psychiatry, 42*(6), 585-590.

Dworkin, G. (1976). Autonomy and behavior control. *Hastings Center Report, 6,* 23-28.

Fisher, A. A. (1989). *The process of definition and action: The case of dangerousness.* Unpublished doctoral dissertation, University of California, San Francisco.

Ethical Problems

Forchuk, C. (1991). Ethical problems encountered by mental health nurses. *Issues in Mental Health Nursing, 12,* 375-383.

Garritson-Hunn, S. (1983). Degrees of restrictiveness in psychosocial nursing. *Journal of Psychosocial Nursing, 21*(12), 9-16.

Garritson-Hunn, S. (1988). Ethical decision making patterns. *Journal of Psychosocial and Mental Health Nursing, 26*(4), 22-29.

Garritson-Hunn, S., & Davis, A. J. (1983). Least restrictive alternative: Ethical considerations. *Journal of Psychosocial Nursing, 21*(12), 17-23.

Gaylin, W. (1974). On the borders of persuasion: A psychoanalytic look at coercion. *Psychiatry, 37,* 1-9.

Glaser, B. G. (1978). *Theoretical sensitivity.* Mill Valley, CA: Sociology Press.

Glaser, B. G., & Strauss, A.L. (1967). *The discovery of grounded theory.* Chicago: Aldine.

Goffman, E. (1961). *Asylums: Essays on the social situation of mental patients and other inmates.* Garden City, NY: Doubleday & Co.

Grey, S., & Diers, D. (1992). The effect of staff stress on patient behavior. *Archives of Psychiatric Nursing, 6*(1), 26-34.

Halleck, S. L. (1974). Legal and ethical aspects of behavior control. *American Journal of Psychiatry, 131*(4), 381-385.

Hatton, D. C. (1985). *Health among Native American elders.* Unpublished doctoral dissertation, University of California, San Francisco.

Heifner, C. (1993). Positive connectedness in the psychiatric nurse-patient relationship. *Archives for Psychiatric Nursing, 1*(1), 11-15.

Holly, C. M. (1993). The ethical quandaries of acute care nursing practice. *Journal of Professional Nursing, 2*(2), 110-115.

Jenks, J. M. (1993). The pattern of personal knowing in nurse clinical decision making. *Journal of Nursing Education, 32*(9), 4399-4405.

Johnson, K., & Morrison, E. F. (1993). Control or negotiation: A health care challenge. *Nursing Administration Quarterly, 17*(3), 27-33.

Kittrie, N. N. (1971). *The right to be different: Deviance and enforced therapy.* Baltimore: Penguin Books Inc.

Leininger, M. (1977). Caring: The essence and central focus of nursing. *American Nurses' Foundation Nursing Research Reports, 12*(1), 2-14.

Liaschenko, J. (1989). Changing paradigms within psychiatry: Implications for nursing research. *Archives of Psychiatric Nursing, 3*(3), 153-158.

Liaschenko, J. (1993). *Faithful to the good: Morality and philosophy in nursing practice.* Unpublished doctoral dissertation, University of California, San Francisco.

Liaschenko, J. (in press). Making a bridge: The moral work with patients we do not like. *Journal of Palliative Care..*

London, P. (1977). *Behavior control.* New York: New American Library.

Lützén, K. (1990). Moral sensing and ideological conflict: Aspects of the therapeutic relationship in psychiatric nursing. *Scandinavian Journal of Caring Sciences, 4*(2), 69-76.

Lützén, K., & Nordin, C. (1993). Benevolence, a central moral concept derived from a grounded theory study of nursing decision making in psychiatric settings. *Journal of Advanced Nursing, 18,* 1106-1111.

McCloskey, H. J. (1980). Coercion: Its nature and significance. *The Southern Journal of Philosophy, 18*(3), 335-351.

Monahan, J. (1984). The prediction of violent behavior: Toward a second generation of theory and policy. *American Journal of Psychiatry, 141*(1), 10-15.

104   *Nursing Care in a Violent Society: Issues and Research*

Morrison, E. F. (1990). The tradition of toughness: A study of nonprofessional nursing care in psychiatric settings. *Image: Journal of Nursing Scholarship, 22*(1), 32-38.

Morrison, E. F. (1992). A coercive interactional style as an antecedent to aggression in psychiatric patients. *Research in Nursing & Health, 15,* 421-431.

Morrison, E. F. (1993). Toward a better understanding of violence in psychiatric settings: Debunking the myths. *Archives of Psychiatric Nursing, 7*(6), pp. 328-335.

Olshansky, E.F. (1985). *The work of taking on and managing an identity of self as infertile.* Unpublished doctoral dissertation, University of California, San Francisco.

Outlaw, F. H., & Lowery, B. J. (1992). Seclusion: The nursing challenge. *Journal of Psychosocial Nursing, 30*(4), 13-17.

Rigdon, J. E. (Dec. 24,1994). Companies see more workplace violence. *San Francisco Chronicle*, pp. B 11.

Ruddick, S. (1989). *Maternal thinking: Towards a politics of peace.* New York: Ballantine Books.

Schatzman, L. (1991). Dimensional analysis: Notes on an alternative approach to the grounding of theory in qualitative research. In D. R. Maines (Ed.), *Social organization and social process: Essays in honor of Anselm Strauss* (pp. 303-314). New York: Aldine De Gruyer.

Sclafani, M. (1986). Violence and behavior control. *Journal of Psychosocial Nursing, 24*(11), 8-13.

Shah, S. A. (1977). Dangerousness: Definitional, conceptual, and public policy issues. In B. Sales (Ed.), *Perspectives in law and psychology* (pp. 91- 119). New York: Plenum.

Shah, S. A. (1978). Dangerousness and mental illness: Some conceptual, prediction, and policy dilemmas. In C. J. Frederick (Ed.), *Dangerous behavior: A problem in law and mental health.* (DHEW Pub. No.78-763, pp. 123-136). Washington, DC: The Government Printing Office.

Snyder, W. (1994). Hospital downsizing and increased frequency of assaults on staff. *Hospital & Community Psychiatry, 45*(4), 378-380.

Steadman, H. J. (1972). The psychiatrist as a conservative agent of social control. *Social Problems, 20,* 263-271.

Steadman, H. J. (1980). The right not to be a false positive: Problems in application of the dangerousness standard. *Psychiatric Quarterly, 52*(2), 84-99.

Stilling, L. (1992). The pros and cons of physical restraints and behavior control. *Journal of Psychosocial Nursing, 30*(3), 18-20.

Stone, A. A. (1975). Comment. *American Journal of Psychiatry, 132*(8), 829-831.

Stone, A. A. (1976). *Mental health and law: A system in transition.* (DHEW Publication No. ADM 76-176). Washington, DC: The Government Printing Office.

Strauss, A. (1987). *Qualitative analysis for social scientists.* Cambridge: Cambridge University Press.

Strumpf, N. E., & Tomes, N. (1993). Restraining the troublesome patient: A historical perspective on a contemporary debate. *Nursing History Review,* 13-24.

Tardiff, K. (1984). *The psychiatric uses of seclusion and restraint.* Washington, DC: American Psychiatric Press, Inc.

Watson, J. (1979). *Nursing: The philosophy and science of caring.* Boston: Little, Brown.

Acknowledgments. The author wishes to thank Marsha E. Fonteyn, R.N., Ph.D., and Joan Liaschenko, R.N., Ph.D., for their continual support and critical reviews.

Index

A

Abuser
  of elder abuse, 8
  psychopathology of, 4
Activist research agenda, 13
Acute trauma, in battered women, 44
Adolescents
  homicide committed by, *x*
  pregnancy, abuse during, 10
Adult children, elder abuse and, 8
Advocacy, 1
Alcoholism, in women, 44–45
American Academy of Nursing
  (AAN), policy of, 14–17
American Public Health Association
  (APHA), Public Health Nursing
  section, 16
American Nurses Association
  (ANA)
  Community Health practice, 16
  policy implications, 14–16
Anxiety, in battered women, 25
Arthritis, 7
Association of Women's Health,
  Obstetric and Neonatal Nurses
  (AWHONN), 14
Autonomy, patient. *See* Patient
  autonomy
Avoidance, 74, 78

B

Battered women. *See* Wife-abuse
  chaotic and disordered life of,
    34–36
  children of. *See* Children of
    battered women

defined, 38
nursing intervention, 39
nursing research, 24–25
planning by, 34
shelters for, 31, 35, 38–39, 49
trauma in, 44
treatment strategies, 38–39
violent life of, 37–38
worries of, *xi,* 23–38
Battered Women's Justice Center,
  Pace University, *x*
Behavior control, ethical problems
  with, 92
Beneficence, 92–93
Bioethics, 94
Birth of baby, impact of, 4
Black Women's Health Network,
  15

C

Card sorting, 28
Care, ethics of, 93
Caregiver, elder abuse and, 8
Case review, significance of, 85
Centers for Disease Control and
  Prevention (CDC), 2
Chemical injury, 2
Child abuse
  defined, 4–5
  incidence of, 5
  National Incidence Study
    (NIS-1), 5
  nursing research, 11–12
  prevention programs *See*
    Hawaii's Healthy Start
    Program
  reduction strategies, 55
  treatment strategies, 5–6, 16

Child Abuse Prevention and
Treatment Act, 4
Childhood history, significance of,
6
Child maltreatment. *See* Child
abuse
Child neglect
defined, 4–5
treatment services, 5
Children, generally
abuse of. *See* Child abuse
of battered women. *See* Children
of battered women
destruction of, *x*
family violence and, 4
Children of battered women
chaotic and disorderly life of,
34–36
mothers' worries about, *xi,* 23,
36–38
nursing intervention, 37
psychological problems of, 11
research study, 24–36
response of, 23
safety of, *xi,* 31–34
treatment programs, 39
violence in, 37
Children's Defense Fund, 16
Chronic pelvic pain, 7
Chronic trauma, in battered women,
44
Civil Rights laws, domestic
violence, *x*
Coercion, 92
Community mental health centers,
49
Comparative analysis, 96
Compensatory Model, wife-abuse
and, 46
Connectedness nurses, 103
Conservatorship, 94
Consultations, significance of, 85

Control, in nurse–patient relationship, 103
Countertransference
CTR I/CTR II research, 79–84
impact of, 76–78
typology of, 78–79
vicarious traumatization and, 71
Coworkers, nurse relationships
with, 103
"Culture of violence," nursing
response to, *xi*
Cycle of violence, 4

D

Dangerous mentally ill, 92
Dangerousness, psychiatric patients
defined, 91–92
ethics and, 94
Death penalty, *x*
Decision-making process, psychiat-
ric nursing, 93
Dependency, elder abuse and, 8
Dimensional analysis, 96
Dissociation, 75
Distrust, in therapeutic relation-
ship, 82
"Doing the right thing," psychiatric
nursing research, 99–101
Domestic violence
incidence of, *x*
laws, inadequacy of, 84
during pregnancy, 3
Downsizing, impact of, 85

E

Elder abuse
classification of, 7
elderly, defined, 7–8
incidence of, *ix,* 8
maltreatment studies, 8

nursing research, 11
risk factors, 8–9
treatment services, 9
Elderly, defined, 7–8
Embarrassment, 51
Emergency department (ED),
female partner abuse research,
10
Emergency Nurses Association, 14,
16
Emotional reactions, 75
Empathic Disequilibrium, 78
Empathic Enmeshment, 78
Empathic Repression, 78
Empathic Withdrawal, 78
Empathy, in vicarious traumatization and, 77–78
Empowerment, 13, 50–52
Enlightenment Model, wife-abuse
and, 46
Ethics, principle-based approach,
93

F

Family Protection and Domestic
Violence Intervention Act of
1994, *xi*
Family violence
child abuse, 4–6
elder abuse, 7–9
homicide and, 3
incidence of, 3–4
response to, 24
spouse abuse, 6–7
Fear, 51
Female partner abuse
incidence of, *ix*
nursing research, 10–11
Feminists, wife-abuse and, 50
Firearms:
deaths due to, 2, 16

possession statistics, *ix*
Flashbacks, 81

G

Gender differences
family violence and, 4
spouse abuse, 6
Gender-politics model, spouse
abuse, 6
Generalized Anxiety Disorder, 25
Grandparents, of abused children,
11
Grassroots movement, 13
Grieving process, 10
Guns. *See* Firearms

H

Hana Like Home Visitor Program,
57
Hawaii Family Stress Center, 57
Hawaii's Healthy Start Program
impact of, 57–58, 67
origins of, 57
purpose of, 55–56
services provided, 59
sources for, 56–57
staffing, 58–59
stages of work with families
assessment/risk reduction,
62–64
high-risk assessment, 64–67
relationship development/
concrete assistance, 59–62
success of, *xii*
Healthy Families America, 56–57
Healthy People 2000, 13, 15, 43
Hearing loss, 7
Holding environment, 55, 65–66
Home visitation programs
child abuse cases, 5

illustration of. *See* Hawaii's
Healthy Start Program
Homicide
female partner abuse, 10
firearms and, 3, 16
incidence of, *ix,* 1
spouse abuse, 6
Homosexual relationships, abuse
in, 6
Hyperautonomic arousal symptoms,
74

I

Injury, generally
intent and, 3
prevention strategies, 14
research, nurse participation in,
13
types of, 2
Intrusive symptoms, 74
Intuition, in battered women, 33
Involuntary commitment, 91
Irritable bowel syndrome, 7

J

Joint Commission on the Accreditation of Hospital Organization
(JCAHO), 15

K

Kempe, Henry, MD, 57
Knives, homicide by, 3

L

Low birthweight infants, 9

M

Machismo attitudes, 6

Mechanical injury, 2
Medical Model, wife-abuse and, 6–
47, 51
Minorities, child abuse and, 5
Models of Helping and Coping,
wife-abuse and, 46–47
Morality, ethics and, 93
Moral Model, wife-abuse and, 46

N

NAACOG. *See* Association of
Women's Health, Obstetric and
Neonatal Nurses (AWHONN)
National Association of School
Nurses, 16
National Center on Child Abuse
and Neglect (NCCAN), 4–5
National Clinical Evaluation Study,
5
National Coalition on Domestic
Violence, 15
National Committee to Prevent
Child Abuse, 56
National Crime Victimization
Survey (NCVS), 2, 4
National Incidence Studies (NIS-1/
NIS-2), 5
National League for Nursing
(NLN), 15
National Research Council, 1
National Women's Health Network,
15
Neglect
of children. *See* Child neglect.
of elderly, 7
Neglect teams, 16
Nightmares, 73
Numbing symptoms, 74
Nurse–patient relationship
ethics of, 102
vicarious traumatization and, 77–
78, 84–85

Index

Nursing Child Assessment Satellite
   Training Scales (NCAST), 62
Nursing education, wife-abuse, 48–
   49
Nursing Network on Violence
   Against women International
   (NNVAWI), 15–16
Nursing research
   child abuse, 11–12
   elder abuse, 11
   female partner abuse, 10–11
   pregnancy, abuse during, 9–10
   psychiatric nursing, 93
   unique perspective of, 12–13

O

Obsession, battered women and,
   25–26
Obsessive Compulsive Disorder, 25
Open-ended questions, 95
Overidentification, 78

P

Passive relaxation techniques, 39
Patient autonomy, *xiii,* 91–92, 96–
   98, 101
Patient noncompliance, 85
Patriarchy, 50
Pelvic inflammatory disease, 7
Perpetrators
   of domestic violence, 84
   of neglect cases, 8–9
Physical abuse
   of elderly, 7
   incidence of, 5
   of women. *See* Battered women
Physical injuries, spouse abuse, 6–7
Physical reactions, 75
Posttraumatic stress disorder
   (PTSD), 72–73
Poverty, child abuse and, 5

Pregnancy, abuse during
   correlates of, 10
   prevalence of, 3, 9–10
Prevention strategies, 13–14
Primary prevention programs
   child abuse, 5
   impact of, 1
Projection, 77
Psychiatric nursing, roles of, 91
Psychoanalysis, 77
Psychoeducational groups, function
   of, 67
Psychological reactions, 75

Q

Quantitative/qualitative analysis,
   13

R

Rape, *ix,* 10, 72, 79
Reciprocity, infant-caregiver
   relationship, 55
Recovery process, 10
Recreational groups, function of,
   66
REM, abnormalities, 75. *See* Sleep
   disturbance
Restraints, use of, 82
Revictimization, 83
Ronald McDonald Children's
   Charities, 56

S

Safety
   battered women's children, 31–
   34
   in psychiatric nursing, 98–99
Secondary prevention, 1
Secondary traumatization, 72
Self-blame, 51

Self-disclosure, 9
Self-protection, 3
Self-system, distortion of, 74
Sentence completion techniques, 28
Sexual abuse
  battered women and, 30
  of children, 11
  female partners, 10
Sexually transmitted disease, 7
Shame, 51
Sigma Theta Tau International, 15
Simultaneous play groups, function of, 67
Sleep disturbance, 73
Spouse abuse, 6. *See* Wife abuse
Stereotypes, of wife-abuse victims, 47–48
Strangulation, homicide by, 3
Stress
  elder abuse and, 8–9
  family violence and, 4
  home visitation programs and, 63
Suicide attempts, of battered women, 44–45
Suicide
  of battered women, 45
  female partner abuse, 10
  firearms and, 3, 16
  incidence of, 1
Support groups, function of, 66
Surveillance systems, 13

T

Temperament, 55–56
Tertiary prevention, 1
Therapeutic relationship
  empathy in, 78
  establishment needs, 91, 99, 101
  vicarious traumatization and, 76
Thermal injury, 2
Transgenerational family violence, 4

Trauma survivors, profile of, 73
Trust, therapeutic alliance and, 82
Type I/Type II (CTR)
  defined, 78–79
  examples of, 79–81

U

Unemployment, impact of, 4
Uniform Crime Reporting (UCR) system, 2
Unit control, maintaining 91–92, 96–98
U.S. Advisory Board on Child Abuse and Neglect, 55
United States Department of Health and Human Services (USDHHS), 15
U.S. Public Health Service, 16

V

Vicarious traumatization
  countertransference, 76–84
  defined, 71
  emotional response to, 72
  evidence for, 72–74
  nursing role, 83
  symptoms of, 75–76
  transference, 76–78
  Type I/Type II (CTR) examples, 78–81
  violence, responses to, 74–76
Victim blaming, *xi*
Victimization
  health problems and, 46
  incidence of, 1
  nursing research, 12
Vigilance, in battered women, 32–33
Violence, responses to, 74–76. *See also* Culture of violence
Violence Against Women Act, *x–xi*

Index 111

Violent psychiatric patients, ethical
  problems with
  overview, 91–94
  research study, 94–101
Violent society, survey of
  data sources, 2
  family violence, 3–9
  homicide, 3
  injuries, categorization of, 2–3
  nursing research, 9–12
Vulnerability, elder abuse and, 8

W

Widowhood, 8–9
Wife-abuse
  injuries, 43–44
  prevalence of, 43–45
  response to
    lack of, 45
    underlying factors of, 46–48
  therapeutic response recommen-
    dations
    empowerment, 50-52
    victim education, 48-50
Work environment
  ethics and, 101, 103–104
  stress research, 73
Workplace, homicide in, 3
Worry, in battered women, *xi,* 25,
  36

Ŝ Springer Publishing Company

WHAT EVERY HOME HEALTH NURSE NEEDS TO KNOW
A Book of Readings

Marjorie McHann, RN, Editor

An anthology of practical, up-to-date readings on home care nursing from leading journals, books, and other sources. Readings were selected for their immediate usefulness to clinicians on topics such as medicare coverage, skilled documentation, clinical management, patient education, quality assurance, and legal issues. A valuable resource for students, practicing nurses, and home care administrators.

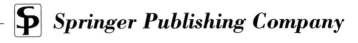

Partial Contents:
Medicare Coverage Issues • Management and Evaluation • The Denial Dilemma • **Skilled Documentation** • Charting that Makes it through the Medicare Maze • Visit Notes • **Clinical Management** • Productivity • Discharge Planning
Patient Education • Successful Client Teaching — What Makes the Difference? • Helping Older Learners Learn • **Quality Assurance Issues** • Patient Complaints • How to Promote Patient Satisfaction • **Legal Issues** • Legal Implications of Home Health Care • Avoiding Professional Negligence: A Review

1995   210pp   0-8261-9130-4   softcover

536 Broadway, New York, NY 10012-3955 • (212) 431-4370 • Fax (212) 941-7842

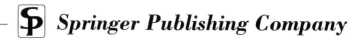

MY FIFTY YEARS IN NURSING
Give Us To Go Blithely

Doris Schwartz, RN, FAAN

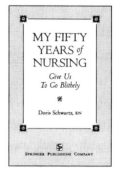

Doris Schwartz's vivid memoirs of her long career as a pioneering public health and geriatric nurse bring readers from the tenements of Brooklyn where Schwartz's patients ranged from Italian immigrants to Mohawk Indians; to the U.S. Army where she spent part of her time as head nurse of an amputee ward and part of the time based in a floating hospital in the Pacific Ocean; to Sweden, where Schwartz visited her rural patients by bicycle; to the Frontier Nursing Service in rural Kentucky where many patients were reachable only by horseback; to a Navajo Indian reservation in Arizona; and to Cornell University and later the University of Pennsylvania, where she spent many satisfying years as a nurse educator, researcher, and writer.

Partial Contents:
The Army Nurse Corps in World War II • Public Health Nursing in Sweden • The Frontier Nursing Service • The Cornell-Navajo Field Health Program • The World Health Organization's "Expert Committee on Nursing" • The Nurse as Primary Practitioner • To the Great Wall of China

1995   224pp   0-8261-8920-2   hardcover

536 Broadway, New York, NY 10012-3955 • (212) 431-4370 • Fax (212) 941-7842

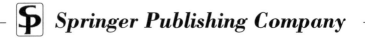

EXPERTISE IN NURSING PRACTICE
Caring, Clinical Judgement, and Ethics

Patricia Benner, RN, PhD, FAAN, **Christine A. Tanner**, RN, PhD, FAAN, **Catherine A. Chesla**, RN, DNSc; contributions by **Hubert L. Dreyfus**, PhD, **Stuart E. Dreyfus**, PhD and **Jane Rubin**, PhD

The long-awaited sequel to Benner's earlier book, *From Novice to Expert*, this book further analyzes and examines the nature of clinical knowledge and judgement, using the authors' major new research study as its base. The authors interviewed and observed the practice of 130 hospital nurses, mainly in critical care, over a six year period, collecting hundreds of clinical narratives from which they have refined and deepened their explanation of the stages of clinical skill acquisition and the components of expert practice.

Contents:
Introduction. Clinical Judgement. The Relationship of Theory and Practice in the Acquisition of Skill • Entering the Field: Advanced Beginner Practice • The Competent Stage: A Time of Analysis, Planning and Confrontation • Proficiency: A Transition to Expertise • Expert Practice • Impediments to the Development of Clinical Knowledge and Ethical Judgement in Critical Care Nursing
The Social Embeddedness of Knowledge. The Primacy of Caring, the Role of Expertise, Narrative and Community in Clinical and Ethical Expertise • Implications of the Phenomenology of Expertise—Teaching and Learning • The Nurse-Physician Relationship: Negotiating Clinical Knowledge • Implications for Basic Education • Implications for Nursing Administration and Practice
1995   416pp   0-8261-8700-5   *hardcover*

536 Broadway, New York, NY 10012-3955 • (212) 431-4370 • Fax (212) 941-7842